Artificial Intelligence in Breast Cancer Early Detection and Diagnosis

Khalid Shaikh • Sabitha Krishnan • Rohit Thanki

Artificial Intelligence in Breast Cancer Early Detection and Diagnosis

Springer

Khalid Shaikh
Prognica Labs
Dubai, United Arab Emirates

Sabitha Krishnan
Prognica Labs
Dubai, United Arab Emirates

Rohit Thanki
Prognica Labs
Dubai, United Arab Emirates

ISBN 978-3-030-59207-3 ISBN 978-3-030-59208-0 (eBook)
https://doi.org/10.1007/978-3-030-59208-0

This Springer imprint is published by the registered company Springer Nature Switzerland AG
The registered company address is: Gewerbestrasse 11, 6330 Cham, Switzerland

Preface

Cancer is a disease that propagates due to the uncontrollable growth of abnormal cells. Abnormal cells perform unusual functions rather than a predefined function within the human body. The growth of normal cells is controllable, while the growth pattern of abnormal cells is recalcitrant. Within a momentary period, the numbers of abnormal cells in the body increase, which in turn creates further complications for proper bodily functions. Cancerous cells can target any organ in a functional body; organs such as skin, lung, and breast are commonly affected. Breasts contain mammary glands and are recognized not only as an important organ but also as a paired structure, which is located on the pectoral region of the chest wall of the human body. They are present in both males and females yet are more prominent in females following puberty. The accessory gland of the female reproductive system's primary function is to produce milk. Breast cancer is a condition in which cells in the breast grow out of control. Various types of breast cancer can originate, depending on which cells are adversely affected.

Our book aims to provide definitive information regarding cancer and breast cancer. The risk factors and prevention of breast cancer are carefully articulated in this book. Information on multiple machine learning and deep learning-based algorithms, along with its working and, usage are thoughtfully discussed in this book. The role of artificial intelligence in the healthcare arena, including medical imaging, is up for debate. Computer aided detection (CADe) system and computer aided diagnosis (CADx) systems along with detection and diagnosis of breast cancer are intricately described.

Finally, deep learning AI models, including their performance within the classification of breast cancer, are introduced and detailed in our effort. We sincerely hope that we can contribute in the eventual technological evolution within the early detection of cancer.

Overview of the Book

In Chap. 1, basic information on cancer and breast cancer are discussed. The various stages and types of breast cancer are beautifully discussed in the Chap. 2. The information on artificial intelligence and various learning algorithms are covered in Chap. 3. In this chapter, the working of various learning algorithms' advantages and limitations are discussed. The role of artificial intelligence and learning algorithms in healthcare sector and medical imaging are covered in the Chap. 4. The information of various stages of computer aided system for detection and diagnosis of breast cancer are covered in the Chap. 5. Finally, Chap. 6 gives a deep learning model along with its performance for the classification of breast cancer.

Features of the Book

- Basic information on cancer and breast cancer
- Various stages and types of breast cancer
- Details of learning algorithms and their role in healthcare and medical imaging analysis
- Computer aided system for detection and diagnosis of breast cancer
- Inclusion of deep learning model for detection and diagnosis of breast cancer

Dubai, UAE

Khalid Shaikh
Rohit Thanki
Sabitha Krishnan

Acknowledgments

Our task has been easier, and the final version of the book considerably better because of the help we have received. I would also like to thank the team at Springer, in particular, Michael McCabe, senior editor, Springer, for their helpful guidance and encouragement during the creation of this book.

Dubai, UAE

Khalid Shaikh
Rohit Thanki
Sabitha Krishnan

Contents

Chapter 1
An Introduction to Breast Cancer

1.1 Introduction to Cancer and Its Treatment

There are many terminologies regarding cancer which are available in literature [1]. According to the American Cancer Society (ACS) [1], it is a disease that disseminates due to uncontrollable growth of abnormal cells. Abnormal cells have an unconventional function rather than a predefined function within the human body. As an example, cells perform multiple functions, such as breathing and walking, while abnormal cells do not perform any of these singular functions; actually they have no useful function but only to harm the body. The growth of normal functioning cells in the body is controlled, while the growth of abnormal cells remains unconstrained. Due to this phenomenon, even for a short amount of time, as the numbers of abnormal cells increase in the body, they adversely affect normal bodily functions.

There is evidence that around 460 to 370 BC, the great Greek physician Hippocrates who is considered the "Father of Medicine" coined the word *cancer* [1] from the words carcinos and carcinoma which describe non-ulcer forming and ulcer-forming tumors. In Greek dialect, cancer was described and imagined by an arthropod of the subphylum Crustacea better known as the crab, due to the fact that the disease spreads in the similar shape of a crab within the human body. The Roman physician Celsus (50 BC to 28 BC) generalized these terms into Latin, while the Greek physician Galen (130 AD to 200 AD) used *oncos* to describe tumors. In general, the crab analogy persists and till today is used to describe malignant tumors [1], while *oncos* describes a special category of cancer under oncology.

K. Shaikh et al., *Artificial Intelligence in Breast Cancer Early Detection and Diagnosis*, https://doi.org/10.1007/978-3-030-59208-0_1

1.1.1 History of Cancer

The history of medicine adequately describes the available information on cancer [2–8]. In the latter part of the nineteenth century, various papyri have described and documented theories on cancer which are made available for extra reading in the below marker.

These documents indicated that the first case of cancer was acknowledged by the papyrus of the great Egyptian civilization. Two of the papyri known as "Edwin Smith" and "George Ebers" have provided exceptional information on it.

The ancient Egyptian mummies with bone cancer were reported in written documents dating around 1600 BC to 2500 BC [9]. Edwin Smith provided information through a cancer survey, while George Ebers provided indulgent information based on procedures for cancer treatment. The information available in the papyri evidences that the ancient Egyptians not only were able to identify malignant tumors but were also able to provide treatment using various methods and medicines.

Pursuant to the historical information on cancer, the second major contributions in the field of cancer are given by Greek and Roman scientists.

Around 1500 AD, Hippocrates and Galen illustrated the natural progression of cancer, including its rudimentary treatments based on their experience and observations. Hippocrates extrapolated the disease with the naming of "carcinoma" (Karkinoma) as "cancer," since the tumor looked like a "crab" and expends like legs of the "crab" from where the tumor is centralized in the human body.

In contemporary medicine, doctors and physicians are persistently observing organs of the human body, to monitor and identify cancer advancements and determine accurate treatment methods.

In the sixteenth century, research on cancer origin was performed by various researchers; by the seventeenth century, the Italian physician Gaspare Aselli discovered the vessel system of the human body and its primary cause of abnormalities in human cells. It was fortunately denounced by Claude Gendron, a French physician who rejected the theory to bequeath a new conclusion regarding the origin of cancer. He was convinced that cancer was a growing mass which was untreatable by medicines and drugs; experiments to validate this theory were performed by two French scientists, physician Jean Astruc and chemist Bernard Peyrilhe, around the eighteenth century. Due to their efforts, various treatments were validated for cancer diagnosis which led to the formation of specialized hospitals.

In the second half of the nineteenth century, the study of abnormal cells and their activity was seamless, due to advancement in microscopes. The process and its findings helped doctors and scientists identify the parameters for cancer origin, and further investigation on cancer tumors revealed dependable information on cancer cells and how these cells were divergent than normal cells. Cancer research and development centers are now diligently working to find a relationship between normal cells and diseased ones.

In the early twentieth century, researchers witnessed a degree of correlation within the cell structures, including the chemistry behind it. Multiple theories developed concerning the treatment of various types of cancers. The initial document regarding the cause of cancer in chickens was dated around 1911 [9]. The primary cause of cancer is chromosomal abnormalities in cells. By 1913, two major publications proclaimed the signs of cancer and the need for a nationwide organization dedicated for its continuous study. These two conclusive reporting established the threat of cancer within the human society. In 1937, the US Congress passed the National Cancer Institute Act. The Act helped create a research institute that was anticipated to develop new theoretical breakthroughs on cancer while promoting R&D in other institutions including coordination of cancer-related projects. In 1971, President Nixon signed another Act to launch a national cancer program, administered by the National Cancer Institute. The primary objective of this institute was not only research but also to create and promote a better understanding of the disease.

1.1.2 Oldest Theories on Cancer

Diverse theories regarding cancer were developed by doctors and researchers [1–9]. The information regarding these theories are listed below.

1.1.2.1 Humoral Theory

The Hippocrates theory was based on the belief that body fluids are made up of four components such as blood, phlegm, yellow bile, and black bile. The imbalance in these fluids causes a disease in the human body. He believed that changes in black bile at the organ site caused cancer in the human body. This theory was recognized as standard up to the Middle Ages around 1300 AD.

1.1.2.2 Lymph Theory

The lymph theory was based on the sensibility that cancer originates due to an imbalance in the lymph fluids. For healthy humans, fluids like blood and lymph continuously move within the body. This theory was validated in the seventeenth century since tumors are created from lymph which is released by the blood.

1.1.2.3 Blastema Theory

The blastema theory was developed by Muller in 1838 and indicated that cancer is made up of cells instead of lymph. Virchow, a dedicated student of Muller, discovered that all cells including cancer cells are derived from other cells.

1.1.2.4 Chronic Irritation Theory

Virchow proposed that chronic irritation was the main reason for causing cancer in the human body. Later, it was discovered that the incremental size of cancer was due to the spreading of malignant cells and not through unbalanced fluids.

1.1.2.5 Trauma Theory

Between the 1800s to the 1920s, researchers were convinced that cancer was caused due to trauma in the human body.

1.1.2.6 Parasite Theory

Till the eighteenth century, doctors and researchers believed that cancer was caused through parasites.

1.1.3 Risk Factors for Cancer

For centuries, scientists and researchers have accumulated data on the exposition of risk factors responsible for causing cancer. They initially believed that cancer was caused due to natural processes like aging; some believed that cancer was hereditary and further investigated human body genetics. Many researchers tried to find chemical links, while some believed that it was caused due to viruses or bacteria. Exhausting all concepts, the "irritation" theory was further developed, and researchers found irritants like coal, tar, and tobacco could cause cancer in laboratory animals. But it was difficult to identify which chemical was the cause.

Although many scientists and researchers have rejected the irritation theory, it was conclusively agreed that it is difficult to identify a single factor that causes cancer.

It is now proven that there are no common factors that can cause cancer; many have tried to find factors that may have a link. Post laboratory experiments, it now believed that some factors such as human lifestyle, surrounding environments, genetics, and many others could be defining factors.

1.1.3.1 Smoking

Cigarette smoking is directly linked as the cause of cancer in humans. One-third of deaths in the United States have been attributed to cancer caused by smoking cigarettes. Lung cancer mainly occurs due to a combination of factors which damage the functionality of multiple organs such as the larynx, oral cavity, and esophagus.

Cigarettes and other tobacco products contain various chemical agents which cause lung cancer. Passive smokers are also at risk due to exposure to tobacco smoke.

1.1.3.2 Lifestyle

Lifestyles that are highly diet dependent play an important role in the cause of cancer. Numerous studies [1] validate the fact that one-third of cancer deaths in the United States happen due to improper diet and lifestyle related factors. Contributing factors are food types, volumes, varieties including processed foods, and a severe imbalance in calories.

1.1.3.3 Genetics

As per definition [1], cancer is a genetic disease. Genes are very small molecules in body cells, which determine everything about a human being. Genes are controlled by genetics and heredity of each cell. In cancer tumors, several gene cells are abnormal, and these abnormal cells foster due to factors such as viruses, uncontrollable cell division, etc. Cancers such as breast, brain, and endometrial are caused by these identified factors.

1.1.3.4 Surrounding Environment

Linking human health conditions to the environment has been identified as another cause. Individuals who have worked in a cigarette smoking environment are at a higher risk of developing lung cancer. Numerous chemicals identified by scientists and researchers which are known to cause cancer are now banned worldwide.

1.1.3.5 Infectious Agents

Viruses cause cancer in the human body. Viruses change the functionality of cells and generate abnormality. For example, the Epstein-Barr virus creates Burkitt lymphoma tumors in African children.

The hepatitis B virus is responsible for liver cancer globally.

1.1.4 Classification of Cancer

Cancers are classified by two ways, cancer origin (tissue) and organ (location in the body where the cancer was developed). Cancer classification based on the type of tissue is recognized as the "histological" type. The international standard for the classification of histological type of cancer is the International Classification of Disease for Oncology [10]. According to this classification, there are different types of cancers which are grouped into six major categories as per below.

1.1.4.1 Carcinoma

Majority of all cancer cases are carcinoma, which refers to a malignant neoplasm of epithelial origin or cancer of the internal or external lining of the body. Epithelial tissues are found all over the body and are present in the skin and in organs including internal part of passage ways, etc. This type of cancer is divided into two major sub-categories such as adenocarcinoma which develops inside an organ and squamous cell carcinoma which originates in the squamous epithelium.

1.1.4.2 Sarcoma

This type of cancer occurs in supportive and connective tissues such as bones, tendons, cartilage, muscle, and fat. This occurs mainly in young adults where painful mass develops on the bone. Sarcoma tumors usually resemble the tissue in which they develop. Examples of this type of cancer are osteosarcoma (bone), chondrosarcoma (cartilage), leiomyosarcoma (smooth muscle), rhabdomyosarcoma (skeletal muscle), etc.

1.1.4.3 Myeloma

This type of cancer forms in particular white blood cells called plasma cells. Plasma cells help you fight infections by making antibodies that recognize and attack germs. Multiple myeloma causes cancer cells to accumulate in the bone marrow, where they crowd out healthy blood cells.

1.1.4.4 Leukemia

Leukemia is also recognized as the cancer of the bone marrow. The word leukemia means "white blood" in Greek. Sometimes, this cancer is called "liquid cancer." This disease often occurs due to the overproduction of immature white blood cells. The abnormal function of these cells creates blood infections. This cancer also affects red blood cells which can cause blood clot formation and fatigue due to anemia. Examples of this type of cancer are myelogenous, lymphatic, polycythemia, etc.

1.1.4.5 Lymphoma

This type of cancer develops in the glands or nodes of the lymphatic system which purifies body fluids and produces infection-fighting white blood cells. Sometimes, this cancer is called "solid cancer." This type of cancer also occurs in various organs such as the stomach, breast, etc.

1.1.4.6 Mixed Types

This type of cancer is a combination of different cancers within one category or from different categories. Examples are adenosquamous carcinoma, mixed mesodermal tumors, etc.

1.1.5 Types of Cancer Based on the Affected Organ

Doctors primarily refer to histological cancers; however the general public is more familiar with cancer names based on the infected organ. The most common human organs in which cancer can develop into are the skin, lungs, female breasts, prostate, colon, rectum, cervix, and uterus.

Listed below are some examples of common types of cancers according to their affected organs.

1.1.5.1 Skin and Lung Cancer

The primary types of skin cancer are basal cell, squamous cell, and melanoma. The first two types of cancer occur on body parts directly exposed by the sun such as the face, ears, and forearm. These are easily detected and removed early, while melanoma which looks like dark moles spread over the skin is the most serious type of skin cancer. It develops in the cells (melanocytes) that produce melanin—the pigment that gives your skin its color. Melanoma can also form in your eyes and, rarely, inside your body, such as in your nose or throat.

Lung cancer detection on the other hand is very difficult because the early symptoms do not appear until it has reached an advanced stage. Symptoms for lung cancer are persistent cough, sputum streaked with blood, chest pain, and repeated attacks of pneumonia.

1.1.5.2 Female Breast Cancer

It has been estimated that in the United States [1], about one in eight women will eventually develop breast cancer in their lifetime, a ductal carcinomas type of cancer. The main risk factors for this cancer are obesity, early menarche (the first occurrence of menstruation), and late menopause. Monthly breast self-examination is recommended as the best way to detect breast cancer early.

1.1.5.3 Prostate Cancer

This type of cancer happens mainly in older men. As men age, the prostate may enlarge and block the urethra. This may cause difficulty in urination or interfere with sexual functions. This condition is called benign prostatic hyperplasia (BPH). The symptoms of BPH may be similar to symptoms of prostate cancer. The symptoms are weak or interrupted urine flow, frequent urination, difficulty in urinating, pain or burning during urination, blood in the urine, and nagging pain in the back, hips, or pelvis.

1.1.5.4 Colon and Rectum Cancer

Colon and rectal cancer is the third most common cancer worldwide. The symptoms of these particular cancers are blood in the stool and a change in bowel habits such as severe constipation or diarrhea. Out of 100 cases, about 70% occur in the colon, and the rest occur in the rectum.

1.1.5.5 Uterus (Corpus Uteri)

The uterus is the sac in a woman's pelvis which allows a baby to develop from a fertilized egg and protects it until birth. This cancer is common worldwide and frequently occurs in women after the age of 60. The symptom of uterine cancer is usually abnormal uterine bleeding.

1.1.6 Cancer Diagnosis Methods

Cancer diagnosis aims to identify the original site of cancer cells and the type of abnormal cells present in it. Cancer can develop in any parts of the human body except the fingernails, hair, and teeth. Here, the site refers to the location of cancer within the body [1]. The body organ in which the cancer develops initially is known as the primary site. These sites provide adequate information, such as the behavior of the tumor, where and which direction it may spread, and what symptoms the tumor can cause. The most common sites in the human body are the skin, lungs, female breasts, prostate, colon, rectum, and the corpus uteri. The secondary site refers to the body part where cancer cells are grown. Cancer is always described by the primary site, even if it has spread to another part of the body.

With the advancement in medical science, symptoms usually indicate the presence of cancer, and these may be observed directly or through various imaging technologies such as computerized tomography (CT), magnetic resonance imaging (MRI), etc. or confirmed by various tests in a laboratory. For example, pink or reddish urine can be caused by an infection in the kidney or cancer. A blood test can confirm a symptom.

A biopsy is preferred to diagnose cancer which involves removal of the affected tissue and examination through a microscope. Tissue sampling is another method that can easily retrieve a tumor from the body surface. If the tumor is inaccessible, then imaging technologies are effective to visually locate a tumor before the biopsy is performed. A histological type of cancer can be easily diagnosed by microscopic examination of the tumor. Biopsies with imaging technologies are widely used for affirmation of cancer within its primary locations and possibly of the location it may spread in.

It is paramount to identify which types of cells are present in a tumor; different types of cancer have different escalation rates that remain dissimilar in nature. Multiple cell types can be present in the same tumor. Thus, once cancer has been confirmed, cell identification is mandatory to know its effect on healthy cells. Cancer cells are said to be different in medical terms [1]. Based on obtained information regarding cells, cancer tumors are rated in different grades: well differentiated (grade 1), moderately differentiated (grade 2), poorly differentiated (grade 3), and uncorroborated (grade 4).

Cancer tumors are further classified according to various stages. Stages are defined on how far a tumor has progressed in the body based on the size of the primary tumor and whether or not it has spread.

Out of all these various diagnostic methods [1], biopsies are preferred by doctors for confirmation. Biopsy provides conclusive information on the type of cancer, its classification, and spread direction including additional information which can help treat it.

1.1.7 Cancer Treatment Methods

Various methods for removing cancer tumors from the body are available in the literature [1, 9, 11]. These methods are listed below.

1.1.7.1 Surgery

Historically doctors knew that cancer tumors can return post-surgical removal. Although benign tumors are not harmful, medical surgeons such as Billroth, Handley, and Halsted surgically removed the entire cancer tumor along with their lymph nodes. Furthermore, Paget discovered that cancer cells can be transferred from the primary site to other locations in the body through the movement of blood. Due to this, the surgery of cancer cells was limited in such a case where the spreading of cells is effective. In 1970, modern imaging technologies were developed in medical science such as ultrasound, CT, MRI, etc. which improved cancer surgery and effectively removed tumors from the body. The introduction of laser technologies helped to remove cancer cells from different organs such as the skin, liver, etc.

1.1.7.2 Chemotherapy

In the last decades of the twentieth century, advancements in nuclear science and chemotherapy radiation theories emerged, and surgeons developed a surgical procedure with chemotherapy radiation for removing tumors from the body. In this treatment, various chemotherapy drugs were used for successive removal of multiple types of cancer tumors from the body [1]. Recently, studies are ongoing to reduce the side effects produced by this treatment and to know how the overall treatment can improve.

1.1.7.3 Hormonal Therapy

In 1878, medical surgeon Thomas Beatson found that breasts of rabbits stopped producing milk after they removed the ovaries [9]. Researchers established that if some parts or vessels from the organ were removed, the growth of cancer was limited and in some cases halted. Recently, new drugs such as LHRH analogs are used for the treatment of breast and prostate cancer.

1.1.7.4 Radiation Therapy

After the discovery of x-ray radiation, scientists actively started using radiation for the treatment of cancer. However, in the early twentieth century, researchers believed that this radiation could “cause” cancer. Now, various radiation therapies are used to kill cancer cells in the body.

1.1.7.5 Adjuvant Therapy

This therapy is used post chemotherapy and surgery to destroy the remaining cancer cells present in the body. This is primarily used for the treatment of colon and testicular cancer.

1.1.7.6 Immunotherapy

A proportion of biological agents are used to control tumor growth in the human body by minimizing neuro signals. This therapy is called immunotherapy. Various biological agents such as interferons, interleukins, cytokines, etc. were developed by researchers in a laboratory for the treatment of cancer tumors. Around 1990, researchers developed agents such as rituximab and trastuzumab which were used for the treatment of cells of lymphoma and breast cancer. Till date, scientists and researchers are developing multiple vaccines to improve the immune system, which could respond positively against cancer cells and tumors.

1.2 Breast Anatomy

Breasts are important organs and paired structures, which are located in the pectoral region of the chest wall of the human body. They are present in all humans, but more developed in the female body. The primary function of breasts in the female body is to produce milk to provide nutrition to a newborn. Hormones such as estrogen and progesterone in the female body are for growth; changes occur in the breast during the menstrual cycle and pregnancy. The breasts are situated on a superficial skin layer on chest muscles which are called mammary glands via numerous ducts to our nipples. There is a dark and circular layer around the nipple called the areola. It is important to understand the normal structure and function of female breasts so that abnormalities can be easily detected and treated. The breast consists of milk glands that produce and supply milk, special ducts that transfer milk from the glands to the nipple, fat, areola, and fibrous tissue. Figure 1.1 shows the inner structure of the female breast [12].

Female breasts are symmetrical in structure and in various sizes such as smaller, larger, higher, lower, or different size from the other depending on the homogenies of the female. 15 to 20 lobes of branching glands are present in fully developed female breasts. These lobes are separated by a connective tissue which eventuates at the nipple. The size, shape, and softness of the breast depend on the fat tissue, which is present in abundance. The special glands in the breast are called tubuloalveolar glands, which are modified sweat glands. Each of these glands ends in a lactiferous duct (2–4 mm in diameter) and opens up through a small hole onto the nipple. Deep into the areola, each duct has a dilated part called the lactiferous sinus, in which milk can accumulate and remain in the nursing mother. Cells that are important in

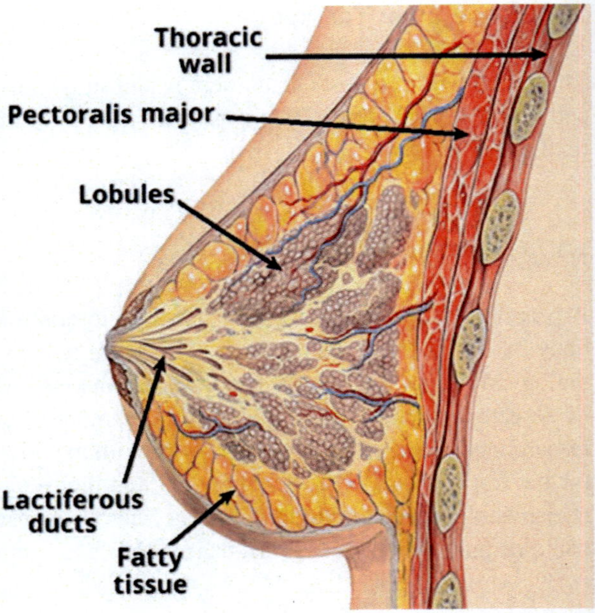

Fig. 1.1 Inner structure of the female breast

contraction movements, called myoepithelial cells, are present in the gland and help in secreting fluids. The nipple and areola are the darker areas of the breast. The nipples contain no fat, hair, or sweat glands. There are many smooth muscle fibers in the breast tissues, which are specially arranged to help the nipple to become erect when stimulated. During puberty, the pigment in the nipple and areola increases, and the nipple becomes more prominent. Within the areola, there are sebaceous glands, sweat glands, and modified mammary glands (better known as Montgomery glands). These glands produce small elevations on the areola surface. The sebaceous glands enlarge during pregnancy and secrete an oily lubricant, for the areola and nipple.

Figure 1.2 shows the arterial supply of the female breast [13]. Arteries carry oxygen-rich blood from the heart to the chest and the breasts, while veins take deoxygenated blood back to the heart. The arterial supply of the breast is from the internal thoracic, lateral thoracic, and thoracoacromial arteries.

1.3 What Is Breast Cancer?

When blood cells in the breast become recalcitrant, the condition is referred to as breast cancer. There are various types of breast cancer, depending on which cells are affected; the three main parts in the breasts are lobules, ducts, and connective tissue. The lobules are where milk is produced, while ducts are channels that carry the milk to the nipple. The connective tissue surrounds and holds everything together. Most cancers happen in lobules or ducts and can spread to other organs of the body

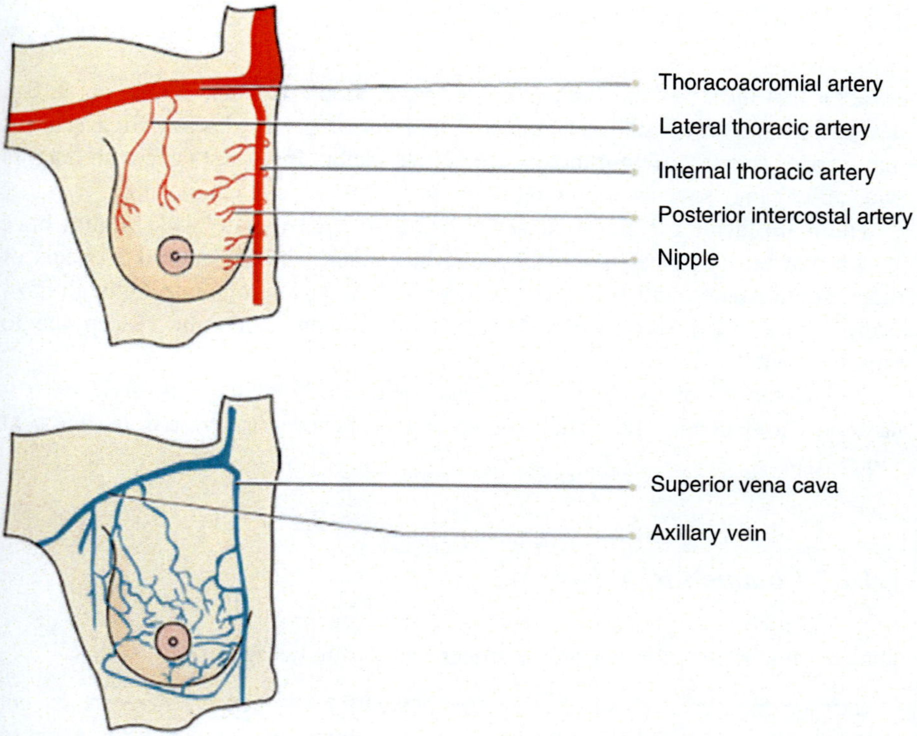

Fig. 1.2 Arterial supply of the female breast

through blood vessels. The most common types of breast cancer are as per below [14]:

- *Invasive ductal carcinoma*: In this type of cancer, the cancer cells are produced outside the ducts.
- *Invasive lobular carcinoma*: In this type of cancer, the cancer cells are produced outside the lobules.

There are other types of breast cancer like external icon medullary, mucinous, and inflammatory breast cancer. Various patients have different symptoms of breast cancer. Some patients may not have all symptoms or any symptoms for that matter. There are however some symptoms or signs of cancer [15]:

- New lump in the breast or underarm
- Thickening or swelling of any part of the breast
- Irritation or dimpling of breast skin
- Redness or flaky skin in the nipple area or the breast
- Pulling in of the nipple or pain in the nipple area
- Nipple discharge other than breast milk, including blood
- Any change in the size or the shape of the breast
- Pain in any area of the breast

1.4 Risk Factors for Breast Cancer

A factor that increases the chances of getting a disease is called a risk factor. But having a risk factor doesn't mean that you are likely to get the disease. Breast cancer may happen due to different factors. Some risk factors for breast cancer are factors you can't change such as getting older or changes of genetic composition.

The main factor for breast cancer is being an aged female [16]. Studies have shown that breast cancer is mostly found in women who are around 50 years or older. Some women will be prone to cancer without any symptoms, although most women have some risk factors, but then all women cannot be susceptible to breast cancer.

Risk factors for breast cancer are common and mostly related to lifestyle, hereditary, and undefined. The details of each risk factor are covered in the next subsections.

1.4.1 Common Risk Factors

The common risk factors for breast cancer are as follows [16, 17]:

- *Being born female*: This is the defining factor for breast cancer. Men can also get breast cancer, but this disease is much more common in women as compared to men.
- *Getting older*: The risk of breast cancer increases when women age. Women around 55 or more are likely to get breast cancer as compared to younger women.
- *Inheriting certain gene changes*: Around 10% of breast cancer cases are generated due to hereditary genes passed from the parent. The inherited mutation of BRCA1 or BRCA2 is the main cause of hereditary breast cancer. A mutated version of these genes can lead to abnormal cell growth which causes cancer. The mutations of other genes such as ATM, TP53, CHEK2, PTEN, CDH1, STK11, and PALB2 may also be a cause.
- *Having a family history of breast cancer*: Women who have blood relatives with breast cancer have a higher risk to contracting breast cancer. But, it is not necessary that women who get breast cancer do not have to have a family history. Women with close relatives such as mother, sister, or daughter with breast cancer are almost at double risk. Women with a father or brother who has had breast cancer may also be at a higher risk. Statistically speaking, about 15% of women with breast cancer have family history.
- *Having a personal history of breast cancer*: A woman with cancer in one breast has a higher risk of developing a new cancer in the other breast or another part of the same breast. Although the risk is low overall, it remains high for younger women with breast cancer.
- *Race and ethnicity*: Caucasian women are slightly more likely to develop breast cancer than African-Americans, although the gap has been closing in recent

years. In women under 45, breast cancer is more common in African-American women, and they are also more likely to succumb at any age. Asian, Hispanic, and Native American women have a lower risk of developing breast cancer. Risk in different groups also varies by the type of breast cancer. For example, African-American women are more likely to have less common triple-negative breast cancer.

- *Being taller*: Many studies have found that taller women have a higher risk of breast cancer than shorter women. The reasons for this are not exactly clear, but it may have something to do with factors that affect early growth, such as nutrition, hormonal growth, and/or genetic factors.
- *Having dense breast tissue*: Breasts are made up of fatty tissue, fibrous tissue, and glandular tissue. Breasts appear denser on a mammogram when they have more glandular and fibrous tissue and less fatty tissue. Women with dense breasts on a mammogram have a higher degree of risk, which is about 1.5–2 times that of women with average breast density. Unfortunately, dense breast tissue can also make it more difficult to identify cancer on mammograms. Several factors can affect breast density, such as age, menopausal status, the use of certain drugs, pregnancy, and genetics.
- *Having certain benign breast conditions*: Women diagnosed with certain breast conditions may have a higher risk of breast cancer. Some of these conditions are more closely linked to breast cancer than others. Doctors often divide benign breast conditions into three groups such as:

  (a) *Non-proliferative lesions* which do not seem to affect breast cancer risk, or if they do, the increase in risk is minor.
  (b) *Proliferative lesions without atypia*: In these conditions, there is excessive growth of cells in the ducts or lobules of the breast, but the cells do not look very abnormal. These conditions seem to raise a woman's risk of breast cancer moderately.
  (c) *Proliferative lesions with atypia*: In this condition, the cells in the ducts or lobules of the breast tissue grow excessively and no longer look normal. Breast cancer risk is about 4–5 times higher than normal in women with these changes. If a woman has a family history of breast cancer and is either hyperplasia or atypical hyperplasia, she is termed as high risk.

- *Starting menstrual periods early*: Women who had more menstrual cycles because they started menstruating early have a slightly higher risk of breast cancer. The increase in risk may be due to longer lifetime exposure to the hormones estrogen and progesterone.
- *Going through menopause after age 55*: Women who had more menstrual cycles because they went through menopause late (after 55) are at a slightly higher risk. The increase in risk may be due to the fact that they have a longer lifetime exposure to the hormones estrogen and progesterone.
- *Having chest radiation*: Women who were treated with radiation therapy to the chest for another cancer when they were younger have a significantly higher risk for breast cancer. This risk depends on their age and when they were exposed to

radiation. The risk is higher for women who have had radiation as a teen or young adult when the breasts are developing. Radiation treatment in older women (after about age 40 to 45) is not known to increase breast cancer risk.

- *Exposure to diethylstilbestrol (DES)*: From the 1940s to the early 1970s, some pregnant women were given an estrogen-like drug called DES because it was thought it would lower their chances of losing the baby or having a miscarriage. These women are at a higher risk of developing breast cancer. Women whose mothers took DES during pregnancy may also be at high risk.

1.4.2 Lifestyle-Related Risk Factors

The lifestyle-related risk factors for breast cancer are as per below [16, 17]:

- *Drinking alcohol*: Alcohol increases the risk of breast cancer. The risk increases with the amount of alcohol consumed. Women who have one alcoholic drink a day have a minor increase in risk as compared with non-drinkers, while women who have two to three drinks a day have about a 20% higher risk than non-drinkers. Alcohol is also linked to an increase in risk of other types of cancer.
- *Being overweight or obese*: Being overweight or obese after menopause increases breast cancer risk. Before menopause, your ovaries make most of your estrogen, and fat tissue makes only a small part of the total amount. After menopause, most of a woman's estrogen comes from fat tissue. Having more fat tissue after menopause can raise estrogen levels and increase your chance of getting breast cancer. Also, women who are overweight tend to have higher blood insulin levels. Higher insulin levels have been linked to some cancers, including breast cancer. The risk of breast cancer after menopause is higher for women who have gained weight as an adult, but the risk before menopause is lower in women who are obese. The ACS [1] recommends you stay at a healthy weight throughout your life and avoid excess weight gain by balancing your food intake with physical activity.
- *Not being physically active*: Evidence is growing that regular physical activity reduces breast cancer risk, especially in women post menopause. The main question is how much activity is needed. Some studies have found that even as little as a couple of hours a week might be helpful, although more seems to be better. Exactly how physical activity might reduce breast cancer risk isn't clear as yet, but it may be due to its effect on body weight, inflammation, hormones, and energy balance. The ACS [1] recommends that adults get at least 150 min of moderate-intensity or 75 min of vigorous-intensity activity each week preferably spread throughout the week.
- *Not having children*: Women who have not had children or who had their first child after age 30 have a slightly higher breast cancer risk. Having many pregnancies and becoming pregnant at an early age reduces breast cancer risk. Still, the effect of pregnancy on breast cancer risk is complex. For example, the risk of breast cancer is higher for about the first decade after having a child, particularly

for hormone receptor-negative breast cancer. The risk then becomes lower over time.

- *Not breastfeeding*: Breastfeeding may slightly lower breast cancer risk, especially if it's continued for a year or more. But this has been hard to study, especially in countries like the United States where breastfeeding for this long is uncommon. The explanation for this possible effect may be that breastfeeding reduces a woman's total number of lifetime menstrual cycles.
- *Birth control*: Some birth control methods use hormones that might increase breast cancer risk. Most studies have found that women using oral contraceptives have a slightly higher risk of developing breast cancer than women who have never used them. Once the pills are stopped, this risk seems to go back to normal within about 10 years. Depo-Provera is an injectable form of progesterone that's given once every 3 months for birth control. Some studies have found that women currently using birth control shots seem to have an increase in breast cancer risk, but other studies have not found an increased risk. Various methods and devices such as birth control implants, intrauterine devices, skin patches, and vaginal rings including commonly used hormones, in theory, could expedite breast cancer growth.
- *Hormone therapy after menopause*: Hormone therapy with estrogen has been used for many years to help relieve symptoms of menopause and help prevent osteoporosis. This treatment has various names such as post-menopausal hormone therapy, hormone replacement therapy, and menopausal hormone therapy. These treatments increase the risk of breast cancer.
- *Breast implants*: Breast implants have not been linked with an increased risk of the most common types of breast cancer. They have been linked to a rare type of non-Hodgkin lymphoma called breast implant-associated anaplastic large cell lymphoma (BAI-ALCL), which can form in the scar tissue around the implant. This lymphoma appears to happen more often in implants with textured surfaces rather than smooth surfaces. If BAI-ALCL does occur after an implant, it can show up as a lump; a collection of fluid, swelling, or pain near the implant; or a change in a breast's size or shape.

1.4.3 Controversial Risk Factors

There are many risk factors that research has shown are linked to breast cancer. But, in some cases, these factors cause breast cancer. The controversial risk factors for breast cancer are as per below [17]:

- *Antiperspirants*: Some of the rumors have suggested that chemicals in underarm antiperspirants are absorbed through the skin, interfere with lymph circulation, and cause toxins to build up in the breast, eventually leading to breast cancer.
- *Bras*: Some of the rumors suggested that bras cause breast cancer by obstructing lymph flow. There is no good scientific or clinical basis for this claim [17], and a

2014 study of more than 1500 women found no association between wearing a bra and breast cancer risk.
- *Induced abortion*: Several studies [17] have provided very strong data that neither induced abortions nor spontaneous abortions have any effect on the risk of breast cancer.

1.4.4 Unclear Risk Factors

Unfortunately research is unclear about how undefined risk factors affect breast cancer risk [17]. The unclear risk factors for breast cancer are as follows [17]:

- *Diet and vitamins*: The possible link between diet and breast cancer risk is unclear. Some research studies [1] have shown that diets do not play a role, while contrarians have found that diet influences breast cancer risk. Studies of women in the United States have not found a consistent link between high-fat diets and breast cancer, although some studies have found a possible link between high-fat diets and a higher risk of dying from breast cancer [1, 17]. Studies looking at vitamin levels in the body have had inconsistent results [1]. So far, there is no strong evidence that taking vitamins reduces the risk of breast cancer [1, 17].
- *Chemicals in the environment*: A great deal of research has been reported, and more is being done to understand possible environmental influences on breast cancer risk [1, 17]. At this time, research does not show a clear link between breast cancer risk and exposure to chemical substances, but studying such effects in humans is cumbersome [1, 17].
- *Tobacco smoke*: Some studies have found that heavy smoking over a long time might be linked to a slightly higher risk of breast cancer. In some studies, the risk has been highest in certain groups, such as women who started smoking before they had their first child [1, 17].
- *Night shift work*: Several research studies have suggested that women who work at night, such as nurses on a night shift, might have an increased risk of breast cancer. Some researchers think the effect may be due to changes in levels of melatonin, a hormone that is affected by the body's exposure to light, but other hormonal imbalances are also being studied [1, 17].

1.5 Prevention Against Breast Cancer

Unfortunately, there is no sure way to prevent breast cancer [17]. There are precautionary measures that might lower your risk, and many risk factors are beyond your control such as being born female and getting older. Other risk factors can be altered and may lower your risk. For women who are known to be at increased risk for breast cancer, there are additional steps that might reduce the risk of developing breast cancer. The various prevention ways which can be performed as per below [17]:

- *Live with a healthy weight*: Both increased body weight and weight gain as an adult woman are linked with a higher risk of breast cancer after menopause. The ACS [1] recommends you stay at a healthy weight throughout your life and avoid excess weight gain by balancing your food intake with physical activity.
- *Be physically active*: Many studies have shown that moderate to vigorous physical activity is linked with lower breast cancer risk, so it's important to get regular physical activity. The ACS [1] recommends that adults get at least 150 min of moderate-intensity or 75 min of vigorous-intensity activity each week, preferably spread throughout the week.
- *Limit or avoid alcohol*: Alcohol increases the risk of breast cancer. Even low levels of alcohol intake have been linked with an increase in risk. The ACS [1] recommends that women who drink should have no more than one alcoholic drink a day. A drink is 12 ounces of beer, 5 ounces of wine, or 1.5 ounces of 80 proof distilled spirits.
- *Other factors that might lower risk*: Women who choose to breastfeed for at least several months may also get an added benefit of reducing their breast cancer risk. To avoid the risk of breast cancer due to hormone therapy, talk to your healthcare provider about non-hormonal options to treat menopausal symptoms.
- *Genetic counseling and testing*: If there are reasons to think you might have inherited a gene change that increases your risk of breast cancer, you might want to talk to your doctor about genetic counseling to see if you should be tested. If you decide to be tested and a gene change is found, this might affect your decision about using the options below to help lower your risk for breast cancer.
- *Close observation*: For women with increased breast cancer risk who do not want to take medicines or have surgery, some doctors might recommend close observation. This approach might include various activities such as frequent doctor visits, early screening of breast cancer, and breast MRI.
- *Medicines to lower breast cancer risk*: Prescription medicines can be used to help lower breast cancer risk in certain women who are at a higher risk.
- *Preventive surgery*: For the small fraction of women who have a very high risk for breast cancer, such as from a BRCA gene mutation, surgery to remove the breasts may be an option. Another option might be to remove the ovaries, which are the main source of estrogen in the body. While surgery can lower the risk of breast cancer, it cannot eliminate it, and it does have side effects.

References

1. What is cancer? American Society of Cancer. Web link: https://www.cancer.org/cancer/cancer-basics/what-is-cancer.html. Last Access: February, 2020.
2. History of Cancer, American Society of Cancer. Web link: https://www.cancer.org/cancer/cancer-basics/history-of-cancer/references.html. Last Access: February, 2020.

3. Hajdu, S. I. (2011). A note from history: Landmarks in history of cancer, Part 1. *Cancer, 117*(5), 1097–1102.
4. Hajdu, S. I. (2011). A note from history: Landmarks in history of cancer, Part 2. *Cancer, 117*(12), 2811–2820.
5. Hajdu, S. I. (2012). A note from history: Landmarks in history of cancer, Part 3. *Cancer, 118*(4), 1155–1168.
6. Hajdu, S. I. (2012). A note from history: Landmarks in history of cancer, Part 4. *Cancer, 118*(20), 4914–4928.
7. Hajdu, S. I., & Darvishian, F. (2013). A note from history: Landmarks in history of cancer, Part 5. *Cancer, 119*(8), 1450–1466.
8. Hajdu, S. I., & Vadmal, M. (2013). A note from history: Landmarks in history of cancer, Part 6. *Cancer, 119*(23), 4058–4082.
9. Sudhakar, A. (2009). History of cancer, ancient and modern treatment methods. *Journal of Cancer Science & Therapy, 1*(2), 1–4.
10. Fritz, A., Percy, C., Jack, A., Shanmugaratnam, K., Sobin, L. H., et al. (2000). In A. Fritz et al. (Eds.), *International classification of diseases for oncology* (3rd ed.). World Health Organization. https://apps.who.int/iris/handle/10665/42344
11. Milestones in Cancer Treatment. CureToday. (2020). Web link: https://www.curetoday.com/search?keywordTerm=Milestones+in+cancer+treatment. Last Access: March, 2020.
12. Breast. Web link: https://en.wikipedia.org/wiki/Breast. Last Access: February, 2020.
13. Mobeen, A., & Manzoor, T. (2014). *Efficacy of combined mammographic and sonographic evaluation of both dense and fatty breast* (p. 11). Lahore, Pakistan: FMH College of Medicine and Dentistry Shadman.
14. What is Breast Cancer? Web link: https://www.cdc.gov/spanish/cancer/breast/basic_info/what-is-breast-cancer.htm. Last Access: March, 2020.
15. What are the symptoms of breast cancer? Web link: https://www.cdc.gov/spanish/cancer/breast/basic_info/symptoms.htm. Last Access: March, 2020.
16. What are the risk factors for breast cancer? Web link: https://www.cdc.gov/spanish/cancer/breast/basic_info/risk_factors.htm. Last Access: March, 2020.
17. Breast Cancer Risk and Prevention. Web link: https://www.cancer.org/cancer/breast-cancer/risk-and-prevention.html. Last Access: March, 2020.

Chapter 2
Types, Diagnosis, and Treatment of Breast Cancer

In the previous chapter, basic information regarding cancer, breast anatomy, breast cancer, and risk factors and prevention of breast cancer have been discussed. In this chapter, various stages and types and treatment methods of breast cancer are discussed. This information on breast cancer is obtained from various Internet sources, cancer-related working agencies, and local hospitals [1–5].

2.1 Stages of Breast Cancer

Once a patient is diagnosed to have some type of tumor or breast tumor, the doctor will then determine the tumor stage to find how far the tumor has progressed. Knowing the cancer stage is the best way to treat and remove it. The American Joint Committee on Cancer (AJCC) launched guidelines for the staging of breast cancer [1]. The staging of cancer depends on the TNM system. The abbreviation TNM stands for size of tumor (T), status of lymph node (N), and metastases (M). After 2018, more measures such as grading of a tumor, the status of various components such as estrogen and progesterone in the tumor, the status of menopause, and overall health of the patient are added in this system. Basic on all these measures, breast cancer is divided into different stages such as stage 0, stage 1, stage 2, stage 3, and stage 4. The details of these stages are described in the next subsections.

2.1.1 Stage 0 and Stage 1

The size of the tumor and place of origin of breast cancer determine the stage of cancer. Carcinoma in situ (CIS) defines stage 0 cancer. The meaning of "carcinoma" is "cancer," while "in situ" means "in the original place." There are three types of

K. Shaikh et al., *Artificial Intelligence in Breast Cancer Early Detection and Diagnosis*, https://doi.org/10.1007/978-3-030-59208-0_2

"carcinoma in situ" such as ductal carcinoma in situ (DCIS), lobular carcinoma in situ (LCIS), and Paget disease of the nipple.

In DCIS, abnormal cells are found in the milk ducts, while growth of abnormal cells in LCIS is detected in the lobules. In stage 0 breast cancer, abnormal cells have not spread outside of the ducts or lobules into the surrounding breast tissue. This type of breast cancer is easily treatable but if untreated can spread into the surrounding breast tissue. Cancer is evident in stage 1 breast cancer, but it is controlled within the area where it begins. Stage 1 breast cancer is divided into two types such as 1A and 1B based on the difference in the size of the tumor and the lymph nodes where abnormal cells are presented. If the size of tumor cells is less than 2 cm and has not spread to the lymph nodes, then this tumor is classified as stage 1A breast cancer tumor. In stage 1B, lymph nodes have small clusters of abnormal cells with an approximated size of the width of a grain of rice. Similar to stage 0, stage 1 breast cancer is easily detected and treatable.

2.1.2 Stage 2

In stage 2 breast cancer, the cancer tumor is growing around the lymph nodes or extended nearby lymph nodes in the breast area. Stage 2 cancer can be divided into two types such as stage 2A and stage 2B. The difference between these stages is defined by tumor size and spread of tumor in lymph nodes. Stage 2A breast cancer is identified using the following assumption: (1) less than four auxiliary lymph nodes have been affected by abnormality, and no actual tumor is presented in these nodes of the breast; (2) size of a tumor is less than 2 cm, and less than four auxiliary lymph nodes have been affected by abnormality; or (3) size of a tumor is between 2 and 5 cm and doesn't spread into lymph nodes. Stage 2B breast cancer is identified using the following assumption: (1) size of a tumor is between 2 and 5 cm, and tumor is spread to less than four auxiliary lymph nodes, or (2) size of a tumor is larger than 5 cm, but does not spread to any auxiliary lymph nodes.

2.1.3 Stage 3

In stage 3, the tumor is extended to beyond limit and has invaded nearby lymph nodes and muscles, but has not spread to other organs. This stage is referred to as an advanced stage of breast cancer and is divided into three subgroups such as stage 3A, stage 3B, and stage 3C. The difference between these stages is identified based on the size and spread of tumors within nodes and surrounding tissues. This stage can be characterized either of the following: the tumor can be of any size and has affected nearby four or more than four nodes with maximum nine lymph nodes, or the tumor has a size larger than 5 cm and small clusters of abnormal cells with a width of a grain of rice nearby lymph nodes or a size as small as a lime, affecting lymph nodes near under the arm or the breastbone.

If any size of tumor and cancer has invaded the breast skin or chest wall with evidence of swelling, inflammation, or ulcers, then this tumor is referred to as stage 3B breast cancer tumor. Stage 3B breast cancer may also have invaded up to nine lymph nodes. Stage 3C breast cancer can be characterized as follows: (1) no tumor found in the breast or tumor may be of any size, and cancer may have invaded the chest wall or breast skin with evidence of swelling, inflammation, or ulcers and has also invaded ten or more lymph nodes under the arm; (2) no tumor found in the breast or tumor may be of any size, and lymph nodes extending to the collarbone area were found to contain abnormal cells; or (3) no tumor found in the breast or tumor may be of any size with lymph nodes under the arm and near the breastbone found to contain abnormal cells. Stage 3C breast cancer is further divided into two types such as treatable and untreatable. In the untreatable stage of cancer, a simple surgery is not enough to rid of cancer.

2.1.4 Stage 4

This is an advanced stage of cancer in which tumor has spread to other organs of the body such as the brain, lungs, bones, etc. The tumor at this stage of cancer is incurable and untreatable. Due to modern medical technology, numerous treatments have been developed that can extend the living life of the patient for several years.

2.2 Types of Breast Cancer

Breast cancer is divided into various types such as ductal carcinoma in situ, invasive ductal carcinoma, inflammatory breast cancer, and metastatic breast cancer [1]. The details of these types of breast cancer are given in the next subsections.

2.2.1 Ductal Carcinoma in Situ (DCIS)

This noninvasive cancer is found in the lining of the milk ducts. Abnormal cells have not spread outside of the ducts into other tissues of the breast. It is a stage 0 breast cancer and easily treatable, but if it's left untreated, then it can spread into the other tissues of the breast area.

2.2.2 *Invasive Ductal Carcinoma (IDC)*

In this type of breast cancer, the abnormal cancer cells are formed in the milk ducts and then spread into other tissues of the breast. These cancer cells can also spread to other organs of the body. It also refers to infiltrative ductal carcinoma. This is the most common type of breast cancer occurring in 70–80 cases out of 100 diagnosed cases of breast cancer. This type of breast cancer mostly affects men.

2.2.3 *Triple-Negative Breast Cancer*

The most common types of receptors such as estrogen, progesterone, and HER2/neu gene known to fuel the growth of breast cancer are not presented into cancer tumors. It means that testing of cancer cells is negative for various hormone lab tests for HER2, estrogen, and progesterone. Chemotherapy is wildly used for the treatment of this type of breast cancer. This type of cancer occurs around 10–20% of cases out 100 diagnosed breast cancers. This type of cancer mostly occurs in young females, African-Americans, Hispanics, and/or those with a BRCA1 gene mutation. This type of cancer is more aggressive and difficult to treat.

2.2.4 *Inflammatory Breast Cancer (IBC)*

It is fast-growing breast cancer in which abnormal cells infiltrate the skin and lymph vessels of the breast. In this type of cancer, no tumor or lump can be felt and isolated within the breast. When lymph vessels become blocked by cancer cells, symptoms of this cancer type appear in the body. Symptoms are (a) persistent itching with the appearance of a rash or small irritation; (b) reddish, swollen, and warm breast; (c) breast skin appearing like an orange peel; and (d) occurrence of nipple changes such as inversion, flattening, or dimpling. This type of breast cancer is classified as stage 3 cancer, diagnosed by doctor expertise and biopsy. Various treatment methods such as surgery, radiation therapy, chemotherapy, and hormone therapy are used to remove tumors in this type of breast cancer.

2.2.5 *Metastatic Breast Cancer (MBC)*

Metastatic breast cancer is a stage 4 breast cancer which has spread to other organs such as the lungs, liver, bones, or brain. The spread of cancer can happen through one or more of the following steps: (1) Cancer cells invade nearby healthy cells. (2) Cancer cells travel through the walls of nearby lymph vessels or blood vessels. (3)

Cancer cells are carried by the lymphatic system and the bloodstream to other organs of the body. (4) Cancer cells stop moving as they are lodged in capillaries at a distant location and divide and migrate into surrounding tissues. (5) Cancer cells form small tumors at new locations. Symptoms of this type of breast cancer may vary, depending on how far your breast cancer has spread and what type of tissue the new cancer growth has invaded.

2.2.6 *Other Types of Breast Cancer*

The most common type of breast cancer is ductal carcinoma in situ (DCIS); however, there are other few types of breast cancer seen in the human body.

2.2.6.1 Medullary Carcinoma

Medullary carcinoma accounts for 3–5% of all breast cancer types. This type of cancer tumor shows up on a mammogram but does not always feel like a lump. At times, it feels like a spongy change of breast tissue.

2.2.6.2 Tubular Carcinoma

Making up about 2% of all breast cancer diagnosis, tubular carcinoma cells have a distinctive tubular structure when viewed under a microscope. It is usually found through a mammogram and is a collection of cells that can feel like a spongy area of breast tissue rather than a lump. Typically this type of breast cancer is found in women aged 50 and above and usually responds well to hormone therapy.

2.2.6.3 Mucinous Carcinoma (Colloid)

Mucinous carcinoma represents approximately 1–2% of all breast cancers. The main differentiating features are mucus production and cells that are poorly defined. It also has a favorable prognosis in most cases.

2.2.6.4 Paget Disease of the Breast or Nipple

This condition (also known as mammary Paget disease) is a rare type of cancer affecting the skin of the nipple and often the areola, which is the darker circle of skin around the nipple. Most people with Paget disease evident on the nipple also have one or more tumors inside the same breast, generally, either ductal carcinoma in situ or invasive breast cancer (1–3). Paget disease is frequently misdiagnosed at first because the first noticeable symptoms can easily be confused with more common skin conditions affecting the nipple. Like all breast cancers, the prognosis for Paget disease depends on a variety of factors, including the presence or absence of invasive cancer and whether or not it has spread to nearby lymph nodes.

2.3 Early Detection of Breast Cancer

According to the American Cancer Society, with early detection of abnormal cells in the breast, survival rate is 99% in the last 5 years. Early detection method includes doing monthly breast self-exams, clinical breast exams, and mammograms. Most people have initial symptoms and signs of breast cancer; however, presence of these symptoms does not mean that the person has breast cancer. By performing monthly breast self-exams, you will be able to more easily identify any changes in breast cancer.

2.3.1 Basic Symptoms and Signs of Breast Cancer

The basic symptoms and signs of breast cancer are the following:

1. *Changes in the breast or nipple:*
   - Nipple tenderness or a lump or thickening in or near the breast or underarm area.
   - A change in the skin texture or an enlargement of pores in the skin of the breast.
   - A lump in the breast.
2. *Change in breast or nipple appearance:*
   - Any unexplained change in the size or shape of the breast.
   - Dimpling anywhere on the breast.
   - Unexplained swelling of the breast (especially if on one side only).
   - Unexplained shrinkage of the breast (especially if on one side only).
   - Recent asymmetry of the breasts (although it is common for women to have one breast that is slightly larger than the other, if the onset of asymmetry is recent, it should be checked.)
   - A nipple that is turned slightly inward or inverted.
   - The skin of the breast, areola, or nipple becoming scaly, red, or swollen or having ridges or pitting resembling the skin of an orange.
3. *Any nipple discharge:* It is also important to note that a milky discharge that is present when a woman is not breastfeeding should be checked by her doctor, although it is not linked with breast cancer. Let your doctor know about any nipple discharge, clear, bloody, or milky.

2.3.2 Breast Pain

Breast pain is any discomfort, tenderness, or pain in the breast or underarm region, and it may occur for several reasons. Generally, breast pain is not a sign of breast cancer.

2.3.3 Breast Cyst

A cyst in the breast may feel like a lump, but upon examination, the lump is a small, generally harmless sac filled with fluid rather than a cancerous or benign lump of cells. You may have one cyst or many cysts that appear together.

2.3.4 Breast Self-Exam

Breast cancer can't be prevented, but you can take three important steps to help detect it earlier. Adult women of all ages are encouraged to perform breast self-exams at least once a month. Johns Hopkins Medical Center states, "Forty percent of diagnosed breast cancers are detected by women who feel a lump, so establishing a regular breast self-exam is very important." While mammograms can help you to detect cancer before you can feel a lump, breast self-exams help you to be familiar with how your breasts look and feel, so you can alert your healthcare professional if there are any changes. Below few methods can be used for self-examination of the breast:

- *In the shower:* With the pads/flats of your three middle fingers, check the entire breast and armpit area pressing down with a light, medium, and firm pressure. Check both breasts each month feeling for any lump, thickening, hardened knot, or any other breast changes.
- *In front of a mirror:* Visually inspect your breasts with your arms at your sides. Next, raise your arms high overhead. Look for any changes in the contour, any swelling, dimpling of the skin, or changes in the nipples. Next, rest your palms on your hips, and press firmly to flex your chest muscles. Left and right breasts will not exactly match—few women's breasts do, so look for any dimpling, puckering, or changes, particularly on one side.
- *Lying down:* When lying down, the breast tissue spreads out evenly along the chest wall. Place a pillow under your right shoulder and your right arm behind your head. Using your left hand, move the pads of your fingers around your right breast gently covering the entire breast area and armpit. Use light, medium, and firm pressure. Squeeze the nipple; check for discharge and lumps. Repeat these steps for your left breast.

2.3.2 *Clinical Self-Exam*

A clinical breast exam is performed by a healthcare professional who is trained to recognize many different types of abnormalities and warning signs. This in-office exam will most likely be completed by your family physician or gynecologist at your annual exam, whereas your breast self-exam is something every woman should do once a month at home.

- *A Visual Check of Skin and Tissue:* During a clinical breast exam, your healthcare provider checks your breasts' appearance. You may be asked to raise your arms over your head, let them hang by your sides, or press your hands against your hips. These postures allow your healthcare provider to look for differences in size or shape between your breasts. The skin covering your breasts is checked for any rash, dimpling, or other abnormal signs. Your nipples may be checked to see if the fluid is expressed when lightly squeezed.
- *A Manual Check for Unusual Texture or Lumps:* Using the pads of the fingers, your healthcare provider checks your entire breast, underarm, and collarbone area for any lumps or abnormalities. It is worth noting that some women have breast tissue that appears to be full of tiny fibrous bumps or ridges throughout, known as fibrocystic breasts. Overall lumpy tissue is something your provider will want to note but is unrelated to cancer. A suspicious lump—the type your physician is checking for—is generally about the size of a pea before anyone can feel it in the breast tissue. The manual exam is done on one side and then on the other. Your healthcare provider will also check the lymph nodes near the breast to see if they are enlarged.
- *An Assessment of Any Suspicious Area:* If a lump is discovered, your healthcare provider will note its size, shape, and texture. He or she will also check to see if the lump moves easily. Benign lumps often feel different from cancerous ones, but any lump found will likely need to be examined with further diagnostic measures. It may be helpful to know that lumps that appear soft, smooth, round, and movable are likely to be either benign tumors or cysts. A lump that is hard and oddly shaped and feels firmly attached within the breast is more likely to be cancer, but further tests are needed to diagnose the problem.
- *The Value of Clinical Breast Exams:* Clinical breast exams are an important part of early detection. Although most lumps are discovered through breast self-exams, an experienced professional may notice a suspicious place that fails to register as a warning in the patient's mind.

2.3.3 *Mammogram*

A mammogram is an x-ray that allows a qualified specialist to examine the breast tissue for any suspicious areas. The breast is exposed to a small dose of ionizing radiation that produces an image of the breast tissue. Mammograms can often show a breast lump before it can be felt. They also can show tiny clusters of calcium called microcalcifications. Lumps or specks can be caused by cancer, fatty cells, or other conditions like cysts. Further tests are needed to find out if abnormal cells are present. Women with the age of 40 and older should have mammograms every 1 or 2 years. Women who are younger than the age of 40 and have risk factors for breast cancer should ask their healthcare professional whether mammograms are advisable and how often to have them. Even women who have no symptoms and no known risks for breast cancer should have regularly scheduled mammograms to help detect potential breast cancer at the earliest possible time.

2.4 Diagnosis of Breast Cancer

Breast cancer can be diagnosed through multiple lab tests such as mammogram, ultrasound, MRI, and biopsy.

2.4.1 Diagnostic Mammogram

A mammogram is an x-ray of the breast. While screening mammograms are routinely performed by a doctor to detect breast cancer in women who have no apparent symptoms, diagnostic mammogram is used after suspicious results on a screening mammogram or after some signs of breast cancer alert the physician to check the tissue. The signs may be a lump, breast pain, nipple discharge, thickening of the skin on the breast, or changes in the size or shape of the breast.

A diagnostic mammogram can help determine if these symptoms are indicative of the presence of cancer. As compared to a simple mammogram, diagnostic mammograms provide a more detailed x-ray of the breast using specialized imaging techniques. The ability of a mammogram to detect the breast can depend on tumor size, the density of breast tissue, and the skill of the radiologist in reading the mammogram. Mammography easily reveals breast tumors in older women while less likely to detect breast tumors in women younger than 50 years. This situation arises because younger women have denser breast tissue that appears white on a mammogram.

2.4.2 Ultrasound

A breast ultrasound is a scanning process that uses penetrating sound waves that do not affect or damage the tissue. The breast tissue deflects these waves causing echoes, which a computer uses to paint a picture of what's going on inside the breast tissue. A mass filled with liquid shows up differently than a solid mass. The detailed picture generated by the ultrasound is called a "sonogram." Ultrasounds are helpful when a lump is large enough to be easily felt, and the images can be used to further evaluate the abnormality. Breast ultrasound can provide evidence about whether a lump is a solid mass, a cyst filled with fluid, or a combination of the two. While cysts are typically not cancerous, a solid lump may be a cancerous tumor. The doctor also uses this method to help measure the exact size and location of the lump and get a closer look at the surrounding tissue.

2.4.3 MRI

Various types of imaging techniques are helpful for better diagnostics of breast cancer. If the initial examination of breast cancer is not conclusive, the doctor recommends a breast MRI to assess the extent of the disease. During a breast MRI, a magnet connected to a computer transmits magnetic energy and radio waves (not radiation) through the breast tissue. It scans the tissue, making detailed pictures of areas within the breast. These images help the medical team distinguish between normal and diseased tissue.

2.4.4 Biopsy

A biopsy is a test that removes breast tissue or sometimes fluid from the suspicious area of the breast. The removed cells are examined under a microscope and further tested to check for the presence of breast cancer. A biopsy is the only diagnostic procedure that can determine if the suspicious area is cancerous. There are three types of biopsies such as fine-needle aspiration, core needle biopsy, and surgical biopsy. These methods can find various factors such as the appearance of the tumor, size of it, and location of the suspicious area on the breast for better diagnosis of breast cancer.

Once the biopsy is complete, a pathologist examines the tissue or fluid samples under a microscope, looking for abnormal or cancerous cells. The complete report of the biopsy is sent to a doctor which indicates that the suspicious area is cancerous and provides a full picture of it. The doctor goes through the report and, if necessary, suggests some treatment options. The biopsy report can contain various assumptions like below:

- The report will indicate that no cancer cells are found (means the cells in the lump are benign), but some treatment may be suggested by the doctor to remove these cells.
- The report will indicate that cancer cells are found; further treatment may be suggested by the doctor assigned.
- *In the case of a surgical biopsy*, the results reveal data about the type, grade, and receptor status of the tumor, as well as the distance between the surrounding normal tissue and the excised tumor. The margin, as we mentioned earlier, shows whether the site is clear of cancer cells. (1) **A positive margin** means cancer cells are present at the margin of the tumor. In cases of positive margins, cancer has spread beyond the immediate area. (2) **A negative margin** or clear margin

indicates there are no tumor cells at the margin. That means the cancer is contained in the area nearest to the tumor. (3) **A close margin** means that the space between the cancerous tissue and surrounding normal tissue is less than about 3 mm (0.118 inches).

2.4.1 Lab Tests

If a patient is diagnosed with breast cancer, then the doctor may suggest some additional lab tests to aid in confirmation of cancer. The most common lab tests are the hormone receptor test and HER2/neu test. Results from these tests can provide insight into which treatment methods effectively work on these cancer tumors or cells.

2.4.4.1 Hormone Receptor Test

A hormone receptor is a specialized protein located on the surface of or within a cell. The receptor binds to the female hormones estrogen and progesterone, which flow through the blood. Once bound, the hormone signals the cell to start growing and multiplying. Many breast cancer tumors contain hormone receptors, often in large numbers. When hormone receptors are present, estrogen and/or progesterone can fuel the growth of cancer. Such hormone-dependent cancers often respond well to hormone therapy, which differs from hormone replacement therapy (HRT). If neither estrogen receptors (ER) nor progesterone receptors (PR) are present, the cancer is said to be "hormone-receptor-negative," and hormone therapy would likely be ineffective.

Hormone receptor testing is generally recommended for patients who are diagnosed with invasive breast cancer. If the doctor orders this test, the patient may be asked to discontinue taking any prescribed hormones for some time before the breast tissue sample is obtained. Usually, the sample comes from a biopsy, but the test may also be performed on tissue removed during a mastectomy.

The testing lab typically uses a specialized staining process on the breast tissue sample to see if hormone receptors are present. The technical name for this procedure is an "immunohistochemical staining assay" or an "immunohistochemistry" (IHC). Findings will be included in a pathology report given to the doctor. If the cancer is deemed "estrogen-receptor-positive" (ER+), its cells have receptors for the estrogen hormone. That means that the cancer cells likely receive signals from estrogen to promote growth. About two out of every three breast cancers contain hormone receptors. If the cancer is progesterone-receptor-positive (PR+), its cells have receptors for the progesterone. This hormone could then promote the growth of cancer.

Breast cancer patients who test positive for both estrogen receptors and progesterone receptors usually have a better-than-average prognosis for survival and a complete recovery than those who have no receptors present. Also, the more receptors and the more intense their reaction, the better they respond to hormone therapy. Patients with one type of receptor but not the other may still reap benefits from this form of treatment, but likely not to the same degree. As mentioned earlier, if the cancer is both ER- and PR-negative, it probably won't respond to hormone therapy. Typical response rates to hormone therapy are as follows:

- ER- and PR-positive: 75–80%.
- ER-positive and PR-negative: 40–50%.
- ER-negative and PR-positive: 25–30%.
- ER-negative and PR-negative: 10% or less.

2.4.5.1 HER2/neu Test

Similar to the hormone receptor test, the HER2/neu test looks for a specific kind of protein that is found with certain types of cancer cells and the gene that produces it. The formal name of that gene is the human epidermal growth factor receptor 2, and it makes HER2 proteins. These proteins are receptors on breast cells. In a sense, genes contain the formula for the number and combination of proteins a cell needs to remain healthy and function properly. Certain genes and the proteins they create can determine how breast cancer progresses, as well as how it responds to various types of treatment.

Healthy HER2 receptors are the proteins that help manage how a breast cell grows, divides, and repairs itself. However, in about a quarter of all breast cancer patients, the HER2 gene isn't functioning properly. It makes an excess number of copies of itself in a process known as "HER2 gene amplification." Then these extra genes instruct the cells to make too many HER2 receptors, which is called "HER2 protein overexpression." The ultimate result is that breast cells grow and divide in an uncontrolled fashion.

The HER2/neu test can determine whether the sample is normal or whether it has too much of the HER2/neu protein or an excessive number of copies of its gene. If you have been diagnosed with invasive breast cancer or have had recurrent breast cancer, your doctor may recommend this test. It will help your medical team determine your prognosis, characteristics of the tumor including how aggressive the tumor is likely to be, and the best treatment options. This test is often ordered in conjunction with the hormone receptor test. Typically, the breast cancer tissue sample from a biopsy or the tumor removed during a mastectomy is used.

There are four tests for HER2, and the results of these may appear on your pathology report, which may take several weeks to come back. The first one is the IHC test, which is short for "immunohistochemistry." It looks at whether there is excess HER2 protein in the cancerous cells. A result of 0 or 1+ indicates there is no excess, 2+ is borderline, and 3+ means the cells test positive for HER2 protein overexpression.

The remaining three tests all examine if the cells contain too many copies of the HER2 gene. These tests are:

- The FISH test ("fluorescence in situ hybridization").
- The SPoT-Light HER2 CISH test ("subtraction probe technology chromogenic in situ hybridization").
- The INFORM HER2 Dual ISH test ("INFORM dual in situ hybridization").

There are only two possible results for these three tests: positive, meaning HER2 gene amplification, and negative, indicating the number of HER2 genes is not excessive. In the pathology report, breast cancers with HER2 protein overexpression and HER2 gene amplification are called HER2-positive. This type of cancer often grows faster, spreads to other areas more readily, and has a higher likelihood of recurring versus HER2-negative breast cancer.

2.5 Treatment for Breast Cancer

Breast cancer may be treated by various methods suggested by the doctor. The most famous treatment methods for breast cancer are surgery, radiation therapy, hormone therapy, chemotherapy, and targeted therapy. Some methods are local, targeting just the area of the breast around the tumor, while others are systemic, targeting a specific area of the breast.

2.5.1 Surgery

This is the most common treatment for breast cancer. This removes the tumor and nearby indicated margins. Surgical options may include various methods such as lumpectomy and mastectomy.

- Lumpectomy
  A lumpectomy usually removes the least amount of breast tissue. The surgeon removes the cancerous tumor and a small portion or margin of the surrounding tissue, but not the breast itself. Even though lumpectomy is the least invasive breast cancer surgery, it can still be very effective, and further surgery may not be needed.
- Mastectomy
  In the past, breast cancer surgery often required removing the entire breast, chest wall, and all axillary lymph nodes in a procedure called a radical mastectomy. While radical mastectomies are less common today, there are instances in which this surgery is the best option to treat cancer. If the cancer is detected early enough, there are usually options that will remove cancer while preserving breast tissue. The common options are a lumpectomy (most often followed by breast radiation treatments) and a partial mastectomy. The more common mastectomy procedures are the following:

(a) *Partial mastectomy:* A partial mastectomy requires the surgeon to remove a larger portion of the breast than in the lumpectomy (perhaps a whole segment or quadrant of tissue) to eliminate cancer. Occasionally, the surgeon will remove some of the linings over the chest muscles as well.

(b) *Skin-sparing mastectomy:* This procedure requires removal of the breast, nipple, areola, and sentinel lymph node (or nodes) but not the breast skin. Many women who intend to have breast reconstruction will opt for this procedure.
(c) *Simple mastectomy (total mastectomy):* This surgery requires removal of the breast, nipple, areola, and sentinel lymph node or nodes. It leaves the chest wall and more distant lymph nodes intact.
(d) *Modified radical mastectomy:* This procedure requires removal of the entire breast, nipple, areola, and axillary lymph nodes but often leaves the chest wall intact.

2.5.2 Chemotherapy

It is a drug-based treatment where a combination of drugs is used to either destroy cancer cells or slow down the growth of cancer cells. In this treatment, cytotoxic drugs are given to patients orally or through a vein, and these drugs travel throughout the entire body. Various factors such as the size of the tumor, stage of the tumor, type of tumor, receptor type and its status, number of abnormal lymph nodes, and risk of cancer spread are considered for selection of right chemotherapy drugs. This treatment is commonly prescribed along with other treatment methods such as hormonal and targeted therapies. It can also be used to shrink a tumor before surgery for easier and safer removal. This treatment kills fast-growing cancer cells but can also damage normal cells. This treatment has some side effects on the human body: (a) reduction in red blood cells, (b) affects the cells that produce hair, (c) changes the balance of cells lining your intestinal tract, and (d) affects the nerve cells.

2.5.3 Radiation Therapy

This treatment is also called radiotherapy which uses high-energy rays to kill cancer cells. It affects cells of a body part which are treated with radiation. Breast cancer radiation therapy may be used to destroy any remaining abnormal cells in the breast or affected area after surgery. This treatment is suggested to patients who have DCIS and stage 1 invasive breast cancer. The radiation is used to kill abnormal cells and reduce the risk of cancer occurring in the affected breast area. There are two types of radiation therapy: external and internal beams. In external beam radiation therapy, external beam radiation such as x-ray is applied on a targeted cancerous area of the breast for 2–3 min. In internal radiotherapy, the doctor injects radioactive liquid to target the cancerous area of the breast where cancer originally began to grow and tissue closest to the tumor to kill any possible remaining abnormal cells. This treatment has some side effects and varies from patient to patient. The common side effects are sunburn-type skin irritation of the targeted area; red, dry, tender, or itchy skin; breast heaviness; discoloration, redness, or a bruised appearance; and general fatigue.

2.5.4 *Hormone Therapy*

Hormones like estrogen and progesterone are chemicals produced by glands in the body. These hormones help regulate body cycles, like menstruation. Sometimes these same hormones can cause cancer to grow. The pathologist performs a test on cancer cells to determine if they have receptors that feed on estrogen or progesterone, stimulating their growth. If the cancer cells have these receptors, a pathologist may recommend hormone therapy drugs such as blockers or inhibitors. These two drugs destroy cancer cells by cutting off their supply of hormones. The most common hormone blocker drug is tamoxifen. It blocks the estrogen-shaped openings in the cells, preventing estrogen-fueled cancers from growing. Hormone inhibitors also target breast cancer cells with hormone receptors, but unlike hormone blockers, they work by reducing the body's hormone production. When cancer cells are cut off with a supply of hormones, the tumor then begins to starve and die. This suggestion of this treatment depends on the life stage of the patient. Hormone inhibitor treatment is used in postmenopausal women.

2.5.5 *Targeted Therapy*

This is a more effective treatment that applies to specific cancer cells without damaging normal cells of the breast. Currently, this treatment is used in combination with traditional chemotherapy. Targeted drugs have fewer side effects compared to standard chemotherapy drugs. Targeted drugs are used to block the growth of cancer cells in specific ways. For example, trastuzumab may be given to a woman whose lab tests indicate that her breast tumor has too much HER2. The currently targeted therapy used in practice is monoclonal antibodies which are laboratory manufactured proteins which bind with certain cells of cancer.

References

1. The American Cancer Society. Web link: https://www.cancer.org/. Last Access: February, 2020.
2. Learn about breast cancer. Web link: https://www.nationalbreastcancer.org/about-breast-cancer/. Last Access: April, 2020.
3. National Breast and Cervical Cancer Early Detection Program (NBCCEDP). Web link: https://www.cdc.gov/cancer/nbccedp/index.htm. Last Access: April, 2020.
4. National Cancer Institute. Web link: https://www.cancer.gov/types/breast/mammograms-fact-sheet. Last Access: March, 2020.
5. Cancer Financial Assistance Coalition. Web link: https://www.cancerfac.org/. Last Access: April, 2020.

Chapter 3
Artificial Intelligence and Learning Algorithms

3.1 Artificial Intelligence

An artificial intelligence system is a computer system that can perform tasks that ordinarily require human intelligence. These systems are powered by various learning methods such as machine learning (ML) and deep learning (DL).

3.2 Machine Learning

Machine learning (ML) is one of the applications of artificial intelligence (AI) [1]. The machine learning algorithms provide automatic learning ability of systems. The performance of this system can improve the learning experience without any complicated programming. Machine learning mainly focuses on the implementation and development of a new model based on the computer system and program that can access the information and use this information to learn for them [1]. These algorithms determine a unique feature or pattern in the given input data that helps in making a better decision-making process. These algorithms are mainly used in applications related to the medical image, computer vision, biometric recognition, object detection, automation, etc. [1, 2]. There are three types of machine learning [1, 2] such as supervised learning, unsupervised learning, and reinforcement learning.

K. Shaikh et al., *Artificial Intelligence in Breast Cancer Early Detection and Diagnosis*, https://doi.org/10.1007/978-3-030-59208-0_3

3.2.1 *Supervised Learning*

This type of learning is mainly used in real-time applications and practical approach. In this learning, the model tries to learn information from the previous experience of information that is given to it.

In this learning, the input (x) and output (y) are determined by an algorithm that gives mapping function (f) from the input to the output as shown below:

$$y = f(x) \quad (3.1)$$

Classification and regression problems are the two main areas where supervised learning is useful. The classification problem is where the output is a specific value, group, or category, for example, "cat" or "dog." The regression problem is where the output is a continuous value or real value, for example, temperature or currency. There are dozens of algorithms developed for supervised learning, and each of them uses various methodologies to predict the value of the output [4].

3.2.2 *Unsupervised Learning*

In unsupervised learning, the algorithms try to discover a unique pattern or feature themselves without the knowledge of previous experience. Mathematically, this type of learning is where the model has input (x) but does not have a corresponding output. This type of learning is called unsupervised because the machine or system itself finds the answer of the input and the correct output is not given. The algorithms based on unsupervised learning are used in problems related to association and clustering.

3.2.3 *Reinforcement Learning*

In this type of learning, a machine or system takes a particular action to maximize output for a given input. It uses various software and algorithms to find the best possible output or behavior of the machine for a given input task.

No machine learning algorithm fits all requirements of real-time applications. Therefore, finding the right algorithms is a challenging task, and it is a trial and error method. To solve this, researchers [1–5] suggest that the selection of algorithms can be determined depending on the size of the input data, the nature of input data, and what type of output is required from the given input data. Thus, in practice, machines are used as reinforcement learning. It exposes to the platform where it continuously trains itself to predict the better output. In real-time applications related to machine learning, multimedia information such as images, videos, speech signals, etc. are

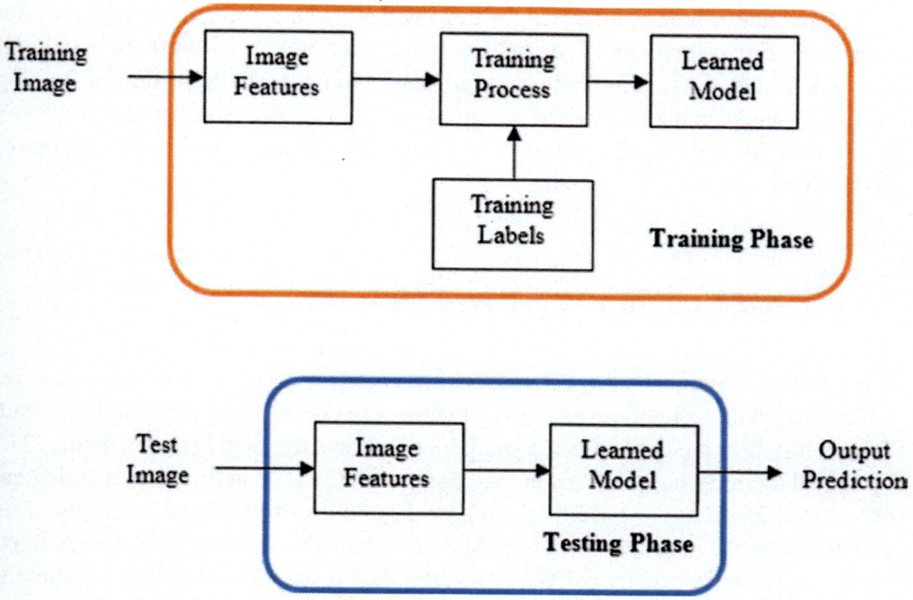

Fig. 3.1 Steps of machine learning algorithm

used as input data. The image related to machine learning applications is very famous in the research community due to its simple visualization and ease of understanding [6]. The basic steps of the machine learning algorithm for image processing are given in Fig. 3.1. This algorithm is working in two phases such as the training phase and testing phase. In the training phase, the model learns unique features or patterns from the input image. While in the testing phase, the model gives the specific output based on learner features or patterns. The features or patterns of the image may be edges, a region of interests, etc. which extract using various feature extraction methods. The selection of extraction methods depends on the type of input image and the specific output of the model.

3.3 Supervised Learning Algorithms

In this type of algorithms, prior knowledge of the dataset is essentially required for the testing of algorithms. This knowledge of the dataset must be gathered by the analyst. The steps in this algorithm are [7]:

- Identifying the training areas for each class of input data.
- Identifying signatures (mean, variance, covariance, etc.).
- All data are then classified.
- Finally, mapping the input class is done.

The main advantage of these algorithms is that it can detect errors during evaluation and correct the detected error. The main disadvantage of these algorithms is that it is a time-consuming and costly process. Moreover, the selection of training dataset depends on the researcher, scientists, or analyst. The quality of dataset again depends on its selection procedure. Thus, these algorithms introduced human error in their performance.

3.3.1 Statistical Learning-Based Algorithms

The statistical learning-based classifiers are based on some mathematics theories which deal to find a relationship between classes to predict some meaningful output. These classifiers are applied to the smaller size of datasets with lower attributes. The statistical learning-based classifiers are not preferable for satellite image classification due to large data of satellite imagery. Examples of statistical learning-based classifiers are the minimum distance (MD), Mahalanobis distance (MhD), and maximum likelihood classifier (MXL) [8]. A detailed discussion of these classifiers is beautifully covered by Lillesand and Keifer [9]. The MXL is widely used for image classification and based on the probability theory of Bayesian. It uses an array of dataset patterns and the covariance matrix of the Gaussian distributed dataset to give the probability of the input dataset. There are lots of limitations of this classifier such as accurate estimation of mean and covariance values of the input dataset, instability in an inverse matrix of covariance between two test image bands, and inapplicability for datasets which have not distributed normally. Table 3.1 summarizes the advantages and limitations of statistical learning-based classifiers [8] [9].

The limitations of statistical learning-based classifiers are applicable for a smaller size of the dataset and less accurate dataset which can be interpreted by machine learning-based classifiers. Machine learning-based classifiers such as an artificial neural network (ANN), nearest neighbors (NN), naïve Bayes (NB), support vector machine (SVM), discriminant analysis (DA), and convolutional neural network (CNN) are mostly applied for image classification and have better performance compared to statistical learning-based classifiers. A brief description of machine learning-based classifiers is covered and detailed in upcoming subsections.

Table 3.1 Advantages and limitations of statistical learning-based classifiers

Classifier	Advantages	Limitations
MD	Simple to implement and fast computational time	Only calculates the mean value of the input dataset and not applicable to a large-size of the dataset
MhD	Simple to implement and fast computational time	Only calculates the mean value of the input dataset and not applicable to a large-size of the dataset
MXL	Simple to implement and done sub-pixel-based classification	Higher computational time and not applicable for large size of the dataset

3.3.2 *Nearest Neighbors (NN) Algorithm*

Nearest neighbors algorithm is one of the famous machine learning algorithms which are used for image classification. It classified the disease portion in the medical image based on the input dataset of their nearest neighbors in the image dataset. It predicts that objects near to each other have similar characteristics. It is a non-parametric algorithm that does not require any assumption for the distribution of the input dataset. It requires some prior knowledge of the input image dataset for the identification of important attributes. For easy understanding of this algorithm, below example is given.

Two datasets are spread in a two-dimensional space which is shown in Fig. 3.2. We need to find a class of data with a plus sign. Data with the plus sign may be class 1 or class 2 and nothing else. The NN algorithm is used to calculate mean values of nearest neighbors in the dataset, and this calculation depends on the value of K. So, sometimes this algorithm is known as the K-nearest neighbor algorithm. Let K have a value of 4. Here, we make a circle of 4 values near to each on the plane. The four closest points in the data with a plus sign are all class 1 data. Hence, it decides that data with a plus sign belong to class 1. The key point in the KNN algorithm is that choice of constant parameter K is very important for proper output.

The steps for nearest neighbors (NN) algorithm are as follows:

1. Let x be several input training dataset and y be an unknown output.
2. Store values of training dataset in terms of arrays, and compute the means of each value of the training set.
3. Calculate the Euclidean distance between each means of the training set. Then, make a set of values y of K smallest distances obtained.
4. Repeat step 2 to 4 for the test dataset to find unknown data points which have K smallest distance. Finally, calculate the accuracy of the KNN algorithm for the input test dataset.

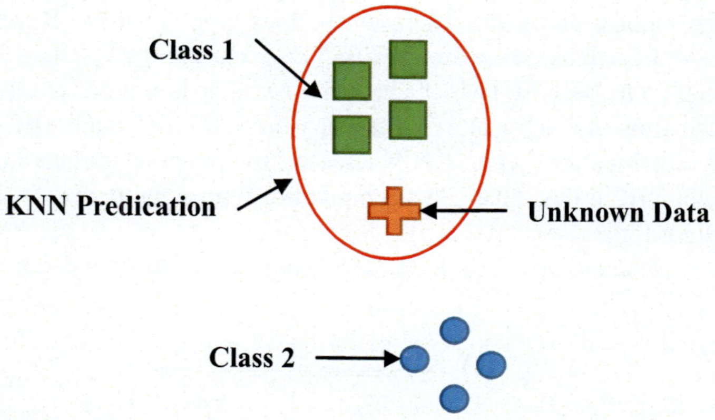

Fig. 3.2 Working of nearest neighbors algorithm

3.3.3 Naïve Bayes (NB) Algorithm

This supervised machine learning algorithm is based on Bayes' theorem with the "naïve" assumption of independent features of each pair of train datasets and test datasets [10]. Given a class variable b and a dependent feature vector a_1, … a, Bayes' theorem has the following relationship for assumption:

$$P(b|a_1,\ldots,a_n) = \frac{P(b)P(a_1,\ldots,a_n|b)}{P(a_1,\ldots,a_n)} \tag{3.2}$$

Using the naïve independence assumption that

$$P(a_i|b,a_1,\ldots,a_{i-1},a_{i+1},\ldots,a_n) = P(a_i|b) \tag{3.3}$$

For all I, Eq. 3.2 simplifies that

$$P(b|a_1,\ldots,a_n) = \frac{P(b)\prod_{i=1}^{n} P(a_i|b)}{P(a_1,\ldots,a_n)} \tag{3.4}$$

For constant input value of P $(a_1,\ldots a_n)$, the classification rule is defined by the below equations:

$$\begin{gathered} P(b|a_1,\ldots,a_n) \approx P(b)\prod_{i=1}^{n} P(a_i|b) \\ \Downarrow \\ \hat{b} = \arg\max_{b} P(b)\prod_{i=1}^{n} P(a_i|b) \end{gathered} \tag{3.5}$$

Here is a maximum a posteriori (MAP) estimation to estimate $P(b)$ and $P(a_i|b)$ for a given input training set. There are various types of naïve Bayes classifiers (NBC) [11–13] such as Gaussian NBC (GNBC), multinomial NBC (MNBC) [12], and Bernoulli NBC (BNBC) which are available in the literature for the assumption of the distribution of $P(a_i|b)$. Out of these classifiers, MNBC and BNBC are used for document classification, while GNBC is used for image classification. The main advantage of NBC is that it has a fast computational time compared to other machine learning algorithms.

In GNBC, estimation of $P(a_i|b)$ is done using below likelihood equation:

$$P(a_i|b) = \frac{1}{\sqrt{2\pi\sigma_b^2}} \exp\left(-\frac{(a_i-\mu_b)^2}{2\sigma_b^2}\right) \tag{3.6}$$

The parameters σ_b and μ_b are estimated using maximum likelihood. The steps for the NBC algorithm are given below [11]:

1. Estimate the densities of the predictors within each class.
2. Model posterior probabilities according to Bayes' rule.
3. Classify an observation by estimating the posterior probability for each class, and then assign the observation to the class yielding the maximum posterior probability.

3.3.4 Support Vector Machine (SVM)

The support vector machine (SVM) is a statistical classification method proposed by Vapnik in 1995 [14–16]. This classifier classifies data by finding a hyperplane (boundary decision) that separates all input data of one class from the other class input data. The best hyperplane for an SVM is the one with the largest margin between the two classes when input data is separated by a linear function. If the input data is separated by a nonlinear function, a loss function is issued to find data on the wrong side of the hyperplane. SVMs use various types of kernel transform to transform nonlinearly separated data into linearly separated data. Three types of kernel functions, polynomial learning machine, radial basis function network (RBFN), and two-layer perception, are commonly used in SVM [15]. In general, the RBFN is used for the training of classifiers as it is more effective and powerful than the other two kernel functions [15, 16]. This classifier effectively classifies input data into two classes, but it can also be used for multiclass classification with error-correcting output codes technique. It is very easy to interpret and proven to be accurate.

A training set is given as

$$T = \{(p_i, q_i) | p_i \in R^n, q_i \in \{-1, 1\}, \quad i = 1, \ldots, n\} \tag{3.7}$$

where p_i is a vector of input values and q_i is a vector of output values.

SVM can generate the desired hyperplane **H** that separates the positive and negative values. If any point of vector x lies on the hyperplane, it satisfies $w \bullet x + b = 0$, where w is normal to the hyperplane and b is a bias function. The optimal hyperplane **H** can be determined by

$$w_0 = \sum_{i=1}^{n} n_i \cdot q_i \cdot p_i \tag{3.8}$$

where n_i is a multiplier that is determined by the SVM algorithm. In Eq. 4.7, points p_i with $n_i = 0$ are eliminated, and those points with $n_i > 0$ are called "support vectors."

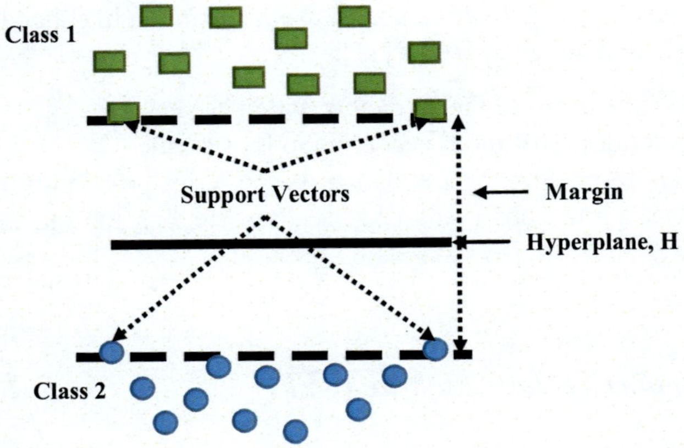

Fig. 3.3 Working of SVM algorithm

Fig. 3.4 Mapping of training dataset using SVM algorithm

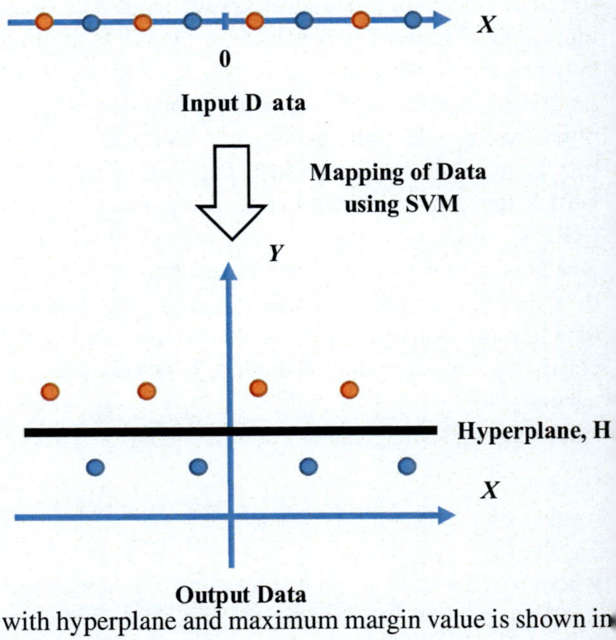

An example of two classes with hyperplane and maximum margin value is shown in Fig. 3.3.

After the training of the algorithm is completed, then hyperplane **H** is determined. Any input data *p* is classified according to the sign value of decision function, which can be given as

$$d(p) = \text{sgn}\left(\sum_{i=1}^{n_i} n_i \cdot q_i \cdot K(p_i, p) + b_0\right) \tag{3.9}$$

where $K(p_i, p)$ is the kernel function that maps the training data to a higher dimensional feature as shown in Fig. 3.4.

SVM has the following advantages: (1) it is flexible for choosing a threshold value for hyperplane, (2) it provides nonlinear transformation, and (3) it provides good capability and eliminates overfitting problem with less computational complexity. SVM also has some limitations: It requires high computational time for training of datasets, and (2) it is hard to understand the structure of the algorithm. Also, the calculation of a separate parameter is not easy due to nonlinear transformation.

3.3.5 *Discriminant Analysis*

Discriminant analysis is a linear algorithm that is used as a dimensionality reduction method in the pre-processing step for image classification. This algorithm is also known as linear discriminant analysis (LDA). The main goal of this algorithm is to convert the input dataset into a lower-dimensional space with reducing computational time and overcome the overfitting problem of classifiers. This method was developed by Ronald A. Fisher in 1936 [17], and it also uses a classifier in some applications such as image classification. The original version of this algorithm was designed for the classification of two classes, and the generalization version of these algorithms for multi-class classification was developed by C. R. Rao in 1948 [18].

Let $A = (a_1,\ldots,a_n)$ and $B = (b_1,\ldots,b_n)$ be samples from two input classes and some abuse of notation $C = A \cup B$. Fisher's linear discriminant is given by the vector w which maximizes [19, 20]

$$M(v) = \frac{V^T P_B V}{V^T P_W V} \tag{3.10}$$

where

$$\begin{aligned} P_B &:= (n_1 - n_2)(n_1 - n_2)^T \\ P_W &:= \sum_{i=1,2} \sum_{c \in C_i} (c - n_i)(c - n_i)^T \end{aligned} \tag{3.11}$$

are the between and within-class scatter matrices, respectively, and ni is defined by $n_i = \frac{1}{n} \sum_{j=1}^{n} c_j^n$. The reason behind maximizing $M(v)$ is to find a direction that maximizes the means of input class while minimizing the variance of the input class in the same direction.

The generalized steps for the LDA algorithm are given below [21]:

- Calculate the D dimensional vectors for the different classes from the input dataset.
- Calculate the scatter matrices in between class (P_B) and within a class (P_W).

- Calculate the eigenvectors and corresponding Eigenvalues for the scatter matrices.
- Sort the eigenvectors by decreasing eigenvalues, and choose N of eigenvalues with the largest eigenvalues to form a $D \times N$-dimensional matrix B where every column represents an eigenvector.

3.3.6 Decision Tree (DT) Algorithm

The decision tree algorithm [22] can be used for solving problems related to regression and classification. This algorithm creates a model that can be used to the classified class using learning decision rules from the training dataset. The understanding of this algorithm is very simple compared to other classification algorithms. This algorithm tries to solve the problem by using the representation of a tree structure. In the tree structure, each internal node of a tree represents an attribute of a dataset, and each leaf node of the tree represented a class label. The basic steps for decision trees algorithm are given below:

- Put the best attribute of the dataset at the root of the tree.
- Split the training set into subsets. Subsets should be made in such a way that each subset contains data with the same value for an attribute.
- Repeat steps 1 and 2 on each subsect until finding leaf nodes in all branches of a tree.

Some advantages of decision tree algorithms are:

- Very easy to implement and understand. Trees can be visualized.
- Requires a very small number of training datasets.
- The construction of the tree is logarithmic in the number of data used to train the tree.
- Able to handle any types of data such as numerical and categorical.
- Able to give multiple outputs.

Some limitations of decision trees algorithms are:

- It creates complex trees that do not give a generalization of data.
- It gives unstable outputs because small variations in the data might change output results.
- Some concepts such as XOR, parity, etc. are hard to understand and to learn because decision trees do not give these concepts easily.

Decision trees are the classifiers used for classification of dataset which has multiple classes in it. The various types of decision tree algorithms available in the literature are ID3, C4.5, C5.0, and CART [23]. ID3 is known as iterative dichotomized 3 and developed by Ross Quinlan in 1986 [24]. The algorithm gives multiple trees for each node of the categorical features of data. C4.5 algorithms are successors of ID3 and convert the trained trees into sets of it-then rules. C5.0 algorithm is the latest version of the ID3 algorithm. CART is known as Classification And Regression Trees and it works similar to C4.5 algorithms, but the only difference is that it supports numerical target variables and does not have any compute sets for tree construction.

3.3.7 Random Forest (RF) Algorithm

The random forest algorithm [25–27] depends on the construction of multiple decision trees. To classify a new class from an input dataset using a random forest algorithm, put the input value of each class on each tree in the forest. Each tree gives a classification, and the average value of trees is given a new class. The random forest algorithm has two stages such as the creation of random forest and prediction of a classifier based on the created random forest. The steps for random forest creation are given below [28–29]:

1. Randomly select p features from the total q features where $p << q$.
2. Among the p features, calculate the node m using the best split point.
3. Split the node into daughter nodes using the best split.
4. Repeat steps 1 to 3 until I no. of nodes has been reached.
5. Build forest by repeating steps 1 to 4 for n no. of times to create n no. of trees.

After the creation of random forest, random forest classification is performed using the below steps:

1. Take the test features, and use the rules of each randomly created decision tree to predict the outcome and stores of the predicted outcome (target).
2. Calculate the votes for each predicted target.
3. Consider the high-voted predicted target as the final prediction from the random forest algorithm.

The main difference between the decision tree and the random forest is that in a decision tree, input training dataset with labels and features is formulated using some specified rules which will be used in classification, while a random forest algorithm randomly selects labels and features to create multiple decision trees and then find average results for each tree.

3.3.8 Linear Regression (LR) Algorithm

As the name indicates, linear regression is a well-known approach for modeling the relationship that lies in between a dependent variable "y" and another or more independent variables that are denoted as "x" and expressed in a linear form. The word linear indicates that the dependent variable is directly proportional to the independent variables. Other things are to be kept in mind. It has to be constant as if x is increased/decreased and then y also changes linearly. Mathematically, the relationship is based and expressed in the simplest form as

$$y = Ax + B \tag{3.12}$$

Here A and B are considered to be constant factors. The goal hidden behind the supervised learning using linear regression is to find the exact value of the Constants "A" and "B" with the help of the datasets. Then these values, i.e., the value of the Constants, will help predict the values of "y" in the future for any values of "x." Now, the case where there is a single and independent variable is termed as simple linear regression, while if there is the chance of more than one independent variable, then this process is called multiple linear regression.

3.3.9 Logistic Regression Algorithm

Logistic regression is a supervised machine learning algorithm used for classification. Though the "regression" in its name can be misleading, let's not mistake it as of regression algorithm. The name logistic regression came from a special function called logistic function which plays a central role in this method.

A logistic regression model is termed as a probabilistic model. It helps in finding the probability that a new instance belongs to a certain class. Since it is a probability, the output lies between 0 and 1. Whenever we are using the logistic regression as a binary classifier (classification done into two classes), we can consider the classes to be a positive class and a negative class. We then find the probability. The higher the probability (greater than 0.5), the likelier it falls into the positive class. Similarly, if the probability is low (less than 0.5), we can classify this into the negative class.

3.3.10 Ensemble Algorithms

Ensemble algorithms are the meta-algorithms that combine several machine learning algorithms and techniques into one predictive model to decrease the variance (bagging) and bias (boosting) or improve the predictions (stacking). The ensemble methods can be divided into two groups:

- The sequential ensemble methods are derived totally from the base learners. And then this is generated sequentially (e.g., Adaboost).
- The primary motivation of sequential methods is mainly to exploit the dependence that falls in between the base learners. The overall performance can be increased and boosted by weighing all the previously mislabeled examples with higher weight.

- The parallel ensemble methods are the base learners which are generated in parallel (e.g., random forest).
- Then there is the basic motivation called the parallel methods which help to exploit independence that falls in between the base learners, since the error here can be reduced dramatically by averaging.
- Most ensemble methods make use of a single base learning algorithm to produce homogeneous base learners, i.e., learners who fall in the same type, leading to homogeneous ensembles.

Few more methods are continuously using heterogeneous learners, i.e., learners that are of different types, and this leads to heterogeneous ensembles. For ensemble methods to be more accurate than any of its members, the base learners should have to be as accurate as possible and even as diverse as possible.

- *Bagging*: The term bagging stands for bootstrap aggregation. One way which is known to reduce the variance of an estimate is by the Average, to average together the multiple estimates. For example, we can train M the different trees on different subsets of the data (which is chosen randomly with replacement) and compute the ensemble:

$$f(x) = \frac{1}{M} \sum_{m=1}^{M} fm(x) \tag{3.13}$$

- *Boosting*: The term boosting here refers to a family of algorithms that are successfully able to convert weak learners into strong learners. The main principle of boosting is to fit a sequence that is made out of weak learners—models that are only slightly better than any random guessing, such as in the form of small decision trees—to the weighted versions of the data. More weight is now given to the examples that were misclassified in the earlier rounds. The predictions are later combined through a weighted majority vote (classification), or it can be a weighted sum (regression) to help produce the final prediction. The principal difference between boosting method and committee method is bagging. This method says it is the base learners who are trained in sequence on a weighted version of the data. And this says it is the base learners who are trained in sequence on a weighted version of the data. Well, the algorithm below describes the most widely used form of boosting algorithm, i.e., called the Adaboost, which stands for adaptive boosting.
- *Stacking*: Stacking is known to be an ensemble learning technique that helps combine the multiple classifications or regression models via a meta-classifier, or it could be a meta-regression. Well, these base-level models are well trained. And this completely depends on a training set, and after that, the meta-model is trained in a way that is based on the outputs that are received by the base-level model as features. The base level is known to be consisting of different learning algorithms, and these algorithms are therefore stacking ensembles that are often considered to be known as heterogeneous.

3.4 Unsupervised Learning Algorithms

Unsupervised learning algorithms are also known as clustering algorithms. These algorithms require minimum input data for analysis compared to the supervised method. In these algorithms, a grouping of the same information in the data is examined. Here, instead of classifying the training user data, the system is allowed to select the mean and covariance of class which will be further classified by the user. The process of classification depends on the system and hence the method called unsupervised classification [30]. The number of classes or clusters can be defined by the user. After classification, the user can assign important information to each cluster for easy analysis. The number of clustering algorithms has been developed by researchers which differ in terms of accuracy and decision-making rules [30]. In all these algorithms used, iterative calculation of input data performs to achieve optimal output for easy decision-making. These algorithms can perform in two steps. The first step is to identify possible clusters within a data or an image. The second step is to estimate a distance measure either between data or on a pixel by pixel basis so that each pixel can be classified into one of the identified clusters [30]. The generalized steps for this classification are as below [30]:

- This algorithm requires the below information such as the radius for the cluster area, merging parameters for a cluster, several pixels evaluated, and the number of identified clusters for the generation of clusters within a data or an image.
- After obtaining a cluster within a data or an image, various labeling is assigned to cluster for proper analysis of data or image.

3.4.1 K-Means Clustering Algorithm

K-means algorithm [30–38] is one of the famous clustering methods for unsupervised image classification. In this algorithm, all the pixels are classified based on their distance from the cluster means [1]. Once the classification is done, the new mean vectors for each cluster are calculated. This process will be performed for a number of iterations until there is no variation in the location of cluster mean vectors between two successive iterations [30]. The main objective of this algorithm is to estimate variation within a cluster. The k-means algorithm performs two steps such as the location of initial cluster centers and after that cluster merging.

The cluster centers generated at the end of the first iteration are taken as the initial cluster center. If x represents the sample space elements of input data, N be the total number of sample space elements, then the mean for data points for the ith cluster in jth dimension is given by Eq. (3.14):

$$c_j = \frac{\sum_{k=1}^{N} x_{kj}}{N} \tag{3.14}$$

The distance of each pixel from all existing clusters is computed, and it is assigned to the cluster yielding the minimum distance. Recalculate the cluster centers using Eq. (3.14). The program terminates once the maximum number of iterations has been reached or by the minimization of the objective function J, i.e., the within-cluster sum of squares as given by Eq. (3.15).

$$J = \sum_{k=1}^{N} x_{kj} - c_{kj}^{\ 2} \tag{3.15}$$

Several measures are available for cluster merging [30, 36–38]. Some of these are listed below:

1. Root mean square (RMS) Euclidean distance for each cluster
2. Matrix of Euclidean distances between cluster centers

The main advantages of this algorithm are that it is easy to implement and that it is a computationally fast clustering method that gives tighter clusters.

3.4.2 Principal Component Analysis

Principal component analysis (PCA) [39–48], also known as Karhunen-Loeve analysis [1, 45, 46], transforms the information in satellite image into new images that provide better interpretation for the original information of satellite image. It compresses the information of the satellite into a few principal component images. The description of the principal component analysis is beautifully described by Schowengerdt [45] and Gonzales-Wood [46]. It transforms the N-dimensional input data X onto a lower k-dimensional ($k \leq N$) value P by maximizing variance or, equivalently, minimizing the reconstruction error [48]. PCA can be represented as

$$P = A^T \cdot X \tag{3.16}$$

where A is formed by the principal components, which are orthonormal and can be obtained from the eigenvalue decomposition of the data covariance matrix. In the machine learning algorithm, PCA is widely used for data reduction for better analysis.

3.4.3 Independent Component Analysis

The independent component analysis (ICA) [49–51] is a computational method of separation data for better clustering. This is done by assuming that the subcomponents are non-Gaussian pixel values and they are statistically independent of each other. ICA is a blind image segmentation method.

3.4.4 Singular Value Decomposition

Singular value decomposition (SVD) [52–54] is a linear algebra method used in many image classification approaches. It is used as a factorization method of linear algebra that describes a rectangular matrix I having rows M and N columns which can be decomposed into a product of three matrices [53].

$$I = USV^T \tag{3.17}$$

In image clustering, SVD is widely used as a preprocessing method and dimensionality reduction of input data. After getting reduced data by SVD, classification of data will be performed [52].

3.4.5 Gaussian Mixture Model

The Gaussian mixture model (GMM) [55–59] is a powerful model for clustering, pattern recognition, and multivariate density estimation [58, 59]. In this model, input data are assumed to arise from a random vector with density

$$f(x) = \sum_{k=1}^{N} p_k \phi\left(x \middle| \mu_k, \sigma_k\right) \tag{3.18}$$

where the p_k is the mixing proportions and ϕ denotes the density of a Gaussian distribution. Generally, the mixture parameters θ are estimated by using maximizing the loglikelihood Eq. (3.18).

$$L\left(\theta \middle| x_1, \ldots, x_n\right) = \sum_{i=1}^{n} \ln \left[\sum_{k=1}^{K} p_k \phi\left(x \middle| \mu_k, \sigma_k\right) \right] \tag{3.19}$$

The main advantages of this algorithm are that it is easy to implement and that it is a computationally fast clustering method that gives tighter clusters.

3.4.6 *Self-Organizing Maps*

A self-organizing map (SOM) [60–66] can generate a visual representation of data on a hexagonal or rectangular grid. Applications include meteorology, oceanography, project prioritization, and oil and gas exploration. A self-organizing map is also known as a self-organizing feature map (SOFM) [64] or a Kohonen map [60, 61]. This algorithm has a set of neurons, which are arranged in a network of a certain dimensionality. The location of any neuron in the network is specified by a position vector v. The weight vector associated with neuron N in the feature map is denoted by W_N. The feature map information follows an iterative process. Initially, the weight vectors are randomly selected, or they are chosen to take advantage of known space in the input data. Then at each time step t, a pattern p, an element of the input data, is chosen at random. The neuron r whose weight value W_r is metrically closet to the pattern p

$$W_r - p = \min_v W_v - p \tag{3.20}$$

is selected. The weight values of all neurons are then changed according to the feature map update rule [31, 32].

$$W_v(t+1) - W_v(t) + et(r,s)\big(p(t) - W_v(t)\big) \tag{3.21}$$

In image processing, the SOM algorithm is used for segmentation and clustering of image and object position changes in the image.

3.4.7 *Hidden Markov Model*

The hidden Markov model has been widely used in various applications such as image segmentation, reconstruction of the image surface, and depth calculation [67]. This model was proposed for the segmentation and classification of various types of images such as MR images and aerial images [68, 69]. Image $I = (i_1,\ldots,i_N)$ where each I_i is the intensity of image pixels. Each pixel is labeled as $X = (x_1,\ldots,x_N)$ where $x_i \in L$ (all possible labels). According to the maximum a posteriori (MAP) criterion, the labeling X' satisfies the below Eq. (3.22).

$$X' = \arg\max_X \left\{ P(I|X,\Theta) P(X) \right\} \tag{3.22}$$

The prior probability $P(X)$ is a Gibbs distribution, and the joint likelihood probability is

$$P(I|X,\Theta) = \prod_j P(I_j|x_j,\Theta_{xj}) \tag{3.23}$$

where $P(I_j|x_j, \Theta_{xj})$is a Gaussian distribution and Θ is an estimation parameter set which is obtained by the expectation-maximization algorithm.

3.5 Reinforcement Learning Algorithm

Reinforcement learning (RL) algorithm [67–69] is a type of machine learning which allows machines to automatically determine the data behavior within a specific manner to improve its performance. The main limitation of this algorithm is that it requires some learning agent. These algorithms are defined for the solution of a specific type of problems. In the problem type, an agent is supposed to decide the best solution that can be achieved based on its current state. When this process is repeated, then it is known as a Markov decision process. Common reinforcement learning algorithms such as Q-learning, temporal difference, and deep adversarial networks are available in the literature [67]. These algorithms should follow the below steps [67]:

- The input state is observed by the agent.
- The decision-making function is used to make the agent act.
- After the action is performed, the agent receives a reward or reinforcement from the environment.
- The state-action pair of information about the reward is stored.

3.5.1 Basics of RL Algorithms

Any RL algorithms are designed to use two common components such as a learning agent and an environment (shown in Fig. 3.5).

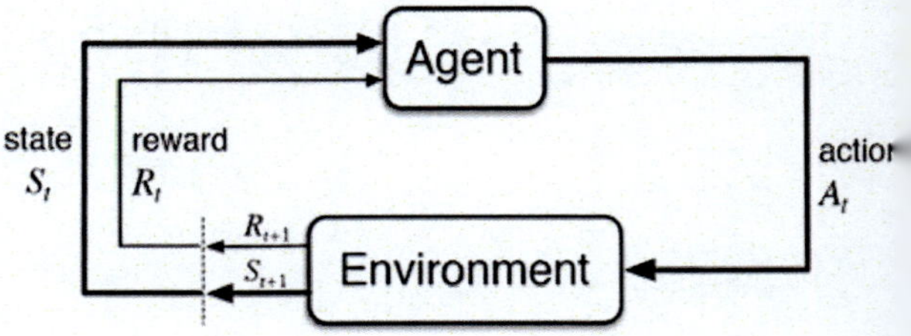

Fig. 3.5 Common components in RL algorithms [70]

The environment refers to the object that the agent is acting on, and the agent refers to the RL algorithm. The environment starts by sending a state to the agent, which then is based on its knowledge to take action in response to that state. After that, the environment sends a pair of next state and reward back to the agent. The agent will update its knowledge with the reward returned by the environment to evaluate its last action. The loop keeps going on until the environment sends a terminal state, which ends with the episode. The common terminologies used in any RL algorithms are as per below [69]:

- *Action (A)*: All the possible moves that the agent can take.
- *State (S)*: Current situation returned by the environment.
- *Reward (R)*: An immediate return sent back from the environment to evaluate the last action.
- *Policy (π)*: The strategy that the agency employs to determine the next action based on the current state.
- *Value (V)*: The expected long-term return with discount, as opposed to the short-term reward R. $V\pi(s)$ is defined as the expected long-term return of the current state s under policy π.
- *Q-value of action value (Q)*: *Q*-value is similar to value, except that it takes an extra parameter, the current action a. $Q\pi(s, a)$ refers to the long-term return of the current state s, taking action an under policy π.

The RL algorithms are classified in various ways such as model-free vs model-based and on-policy vs. off-policy.

- *Model-Free vs. Model-Based*

  The model stands for the simulation of the dynamics of the environment. That is, the model learns the transition probability $T(s_1|(s_0, a))$ from the pair of current state s_0 and action a to the next state s_1. If the transition probability is successfully learned, the agent will know how likely to enter a specific state given the current state and action. However, model-based algorithms become impractical as the state space and action space grow. On the other hand, model-free algorithms rely on trial-and-error to update their knowledge. As a result, it does not require space to store all combinations of states and actions.

- *On-Policy vs. Off-Policy*

  An on-policy agent learns the value based on its current action derived from the current policy, whereas its off-policy counterpart learns the value based on the action obtained from another policy.

3.5.2 Q-Learning Algorithm

Q-learning algorithm is an off-policy, model-free RL algorithm based on the well-known Bellman Eq. (3.24):

$$\upsilon(s) = \mathrm{E}\left[R_{t+1} + \lambda\upsilon(S_{t+1}) | S_t = s\right] \tag{3.24}$$

where E is an expectation and λ is a discount factor. Equation 3.24 can be rewritten in the form of Q-value as per below:

$$\begin{aligned} Q^{\pi}(s,a) &= \mathrm{E}\left[r_{t+1} + \lambda r_{t+2} + \lambda^2 r_{t+3} + \cdots | s,a\right] \\ Q^{\pi}(s,a) &= \mathrm{E}_{S'}\left[r + \lambda Q^{\pi}(s',a') | s,a\right] \end{aligned} \tag{3.25}$$

The optimal Q-value denoted as Q^* can be expressed as

$$Q*(s,a) = \mathrm{E}_{s'}\left[r + \lambda \max_{a'} Q*(s',a') | s,a\right] \tag{3.26}$$

The main goal of the algorithm is to maximize the Q-value. This algorithm works on two iteration methods such as policy iteration and value iteration. In policy iteration, a loop runs between policy evaluation and policy improvement. Policy evaluation estimates the value function V with the greedy policy obtained from the last policy improvement. Policy improvement updates the policy with the action that maximizes V for each of the states. The update equations are based on Eq. 3.24 and keep iterating till convergence.

Value iteration contains only one component which updates the values function V based on the optimal Bellman Eq. 3.25. After the iteration converges, the optimal policy is straightforwardly derived by applying an argument max function for all of the states.

3.5.3 State Action Reward State Action (SARSA) Algorithm

SARSA very much resembles Q-learning. The key difference between SARSA and Q-learning is that SARSA is an on-policy algorithm. It implies that SARSA learns the Q-value based on the action performed by the current policy instead of the greedy policy.

3.5.4 *Deep Q Network (DQN) Algorithm*

Although Q-learning is a very powerful algorithm, its main weakness is the lack of generality. If you view Q-learning as updating numbers in a two-dimensional array (Action Space * State Space), it resembles dynamic programming. This indicates that for states that the Q-learning agent has not seen before, it has no clue which action to take. In other words, the Q-learning agent cannot estimate the value for unseen states. To deal with this problem, DQN gets rid of the two-dimensional array by introducing a neural network. DQN leverages a neural network to estimate the Q-value function. The input for the network is current, while the output is the corresponding Q-value for each of the actions.

3.6 Deep Learning

The first neural network (NN) was introduced by Dr. Robert Hecht-Nielsen who was the inventor of the first neurocomputers [71]. This network is known as an artificial neural network (ANN). He defines a neural network as "a computing system made up of several simple, highly interconnected processing elements which process information by their dynamic state response to external inputs" [71, 72]. This network is mainly used in applications such as big data analysis, person recognition, data prediction, etc. This network is also referred to as a forwarding neural network (FNN). This network uses numbers of neurons which are based on the parallel operation and put in tiers. A simple model for the neural network is shown in Fig. 3.6. The network has mainly three layers, the input layer, hidden layers, and the output layer. The number of neurons or nodes depends on the size of inputs and outputs. Each node is fully connected to its adjacent layers. Two nodes of each adjacent layer are connected by a link with a specific weighting value.

The output of this model (seen in Figs. 3.2 and 3.3) can be given by the below equation:

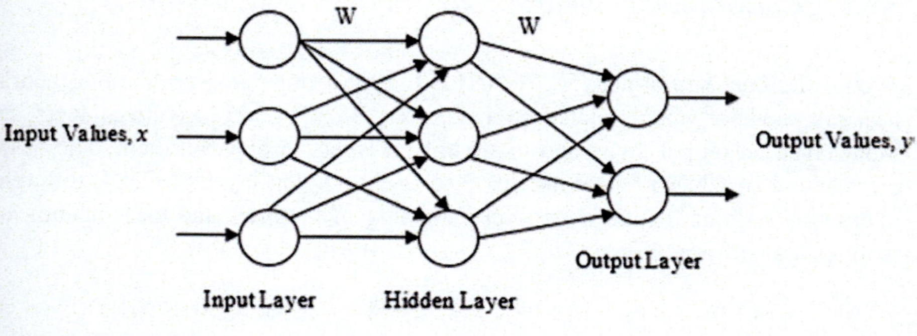

Fig. 3.6 Basic model of artificial neural network (ANN)

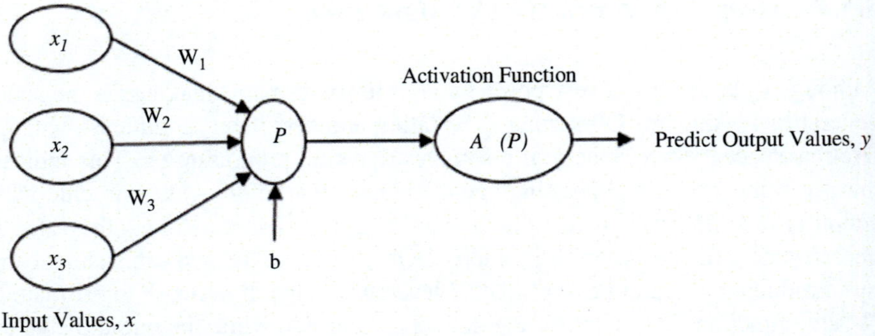

Fig. 3.7 Working of artificial neural network (ANN)

$$y = P + b \tag{3.27}$$

$$P = W_1 \cdot x_1 + W_2 \cdot x_2 + W_3 \cdot x_3 + b \tag{3.28}$$

where x is the input value, W is the weights that are to be learned, b is the bias, and y is the predict output value given by the model. The detailed working of this model is given in Fig. 3.7. The neural network is unable to learn weights for unstructured data such as images and videos. Therefore, activation functions such as sigmoid and ReLU (rectified linear unit) are with the neural network when it is used in machine learning applications. Here, the bias is used for the shifting of activation function for better prediction of data.

A deep learning algorithm is an extension of the artificial neural network. The deep learning algorithm consists of an input layer, several hidden layers, and an output layer. Here, each layer is connected via nodes where each hidden layer gives predicted results based on a prediction of the previous layer. The main difference between ANN and deep learning algorithms is that ANN has one hidden layer, while deep learning algorithms have two or more than two hidden layers. The basic architecture of a deep learning algorithm is given in Fig. 3.8.

3.6.1 Convolutional Neural Network (CNN) Algorithm

A convolutional neural network (CNN) is the most popular deep learning neural network used for image-related applications [73–76]. CNN has three layers, an input layer, an output layer, and many hidden layers in between them. The basic architecture of CNN is given in Fig. 3.9. In the hidden layer of CNN, different operations such as feature extraction, flattening of features, and classification of features are performed.

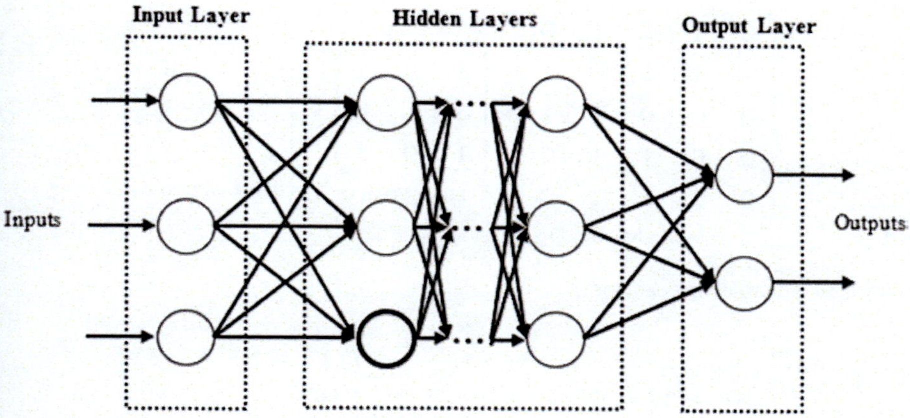

Fig. 3.8 Basic model of deep learning neural network (DLNN)

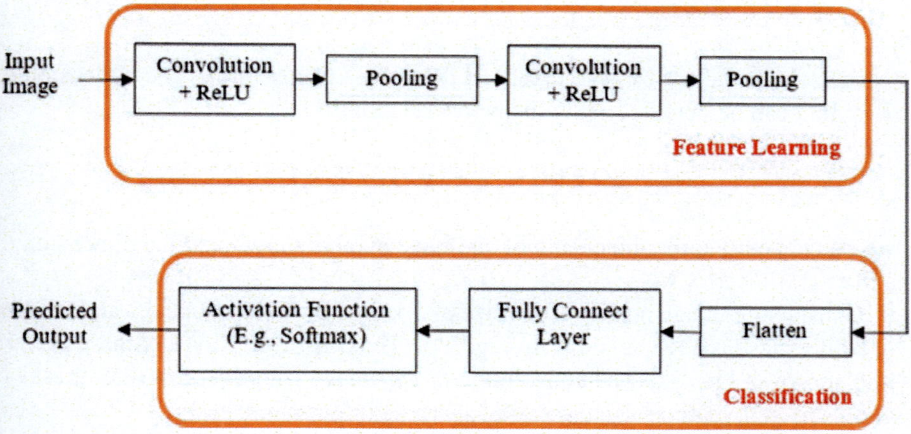

Fig. 3.9 Working of convolutional neural network (CNN)

3.6.1.1 Feature Extraction Operation

The feature extraction operation performs different tasks such as convolution, non-linearity rectified linear unit (ReLU), and pooling. The operation of each task is given below:

- *Convolution*: This is the first step of feature extraction of the input image on CNN. It is a similar process of spatial filtering of the image and gives the relationship between image pixel by obtaining image features using small information of input image. Mathematically, it is the output that uses two input values

$$\underbrace{\begin{bmatrix} 0 & 1 & 1 & 1 & 0 \\ 0 & 1 & 1 & 0 & 1 \\ 0 & 0 & 0 & 1 & 1 \\ 0 & 0 & 1 & 1 & 0 \\ 0 & 1 & 1 & 1 & 0 \end{bmatrix}}_{\textbf{Image Matrix}} \times \underbrace{\begin{bmatrix} 1 & 0 & 1 \\ 0 & 1 & 0 \\ 1 & 0 & 1 \end{bmatrix}}_{\textbf{Filter Mask}} = \underbrace{\begin{bmatrix} 2 & 4 & 4 \\ 2 & 3 & 3 \\ 1 & 3 & 3 \end{bmatrix}}_{\textbf{Convolved Features}}$$

Fig. 3.10 Convolution operation

$$\begin{bmatrix} 1 & 26 & -7 & 35 \\ 16 & -116 & 24 & -9 \\ 26 & -18 & 19 & -50 \\ 101 & 75 & 14 & 45 \end{bmatrix} \xrightarrow{\textbf{Transfer Function}} \begin{bmatrix} 1 & 26 & 0 & 35 \\ 16 & 0 & 24 & 0 \\ 26 & 0 & 19 & 0 \\ 101 & 75 & 14 & 45 \end{bmatrix}$$

Fig. 3.11 ReLU operation

such as the value of image pixel and the value of filter mask. The dimension of output can be obtained using the below relationship:

$$O = (M - f_M + 1) \times (N - f_N + 1) \tag{3.29}$$

where O is output, the dimension of an image pixel is $f_M \times f_N$, and the dimension of a filter mask is $M \times N$.

Consider an image matrix with a size of 5 × 5 with values of 0 and 1 and the size of a filter mask is 3 × 3 as shown in Fig. 3.10. The convolved values of these two are also shown in Fig. 3.6. The convolution of the image with different filter masks is given different features such as edges, sharping information, etc.

Operations like strides and padding are also used after the convolution process for better extraction of the feature. Strides operation is used to shift the value in the image matrix to obtain better features from the input image. Sometimes, the application of a filter to the input image does not fit perfectly; hence padding operation is performed. In this operation some images have 0 values, so that filter works effectively on it.

- *Nonlinearity ReLU*: The nonlinearity ReLU is rectified unit which performed a nonlinear operation on convolved features. It removes negative values in the convolved features (an example is seen in Fig. 3.11). This unit uses various operations such as max, min, mean, etc.

Fig. 3.12 Average pooling operation

$$\begin{bmatrix} 1 & 1 & 2 & 4 \\ 5 & 6 & 7 & 8 \\ 3 & 2 & 1 & 0 \\ 1 & 2 & 3 & 4 \end{bmatrix} \xrightarrow[\text{Filter Mask (2×2)}]{\text{Average Pool with}} \begin{bmatrix} 3 & 5 \\ 2 & 2 \end{bmatrix}$$

- *Pooling*: The process is also known as upsampling or downsampling which reduces the dimension size of each feature. The different types of pooling operations such as max, sum, and average are used in CNN for dimension reduction of extracted features. The example of average pooling is shown in Fig. 3.12.

3.6.1.2 Classification Operation

This operation consists of three different operations such as flatten, prediction of features, and activation function. Flatten is flattening out extracted features from the input image into vector. This vector is fed to a fully connected network such as a neural network for prediction of the input feature vector. Finally, an activation function such as softmax or sigmoid is used to classify the predicted value of the output of the neural network.

3.6.2 Other Deep Learning Algorithms

In the literature, various types of deep learning algorithms are used for research on image-related applications [71]. These algorithms are convolutional neural networks (CNN), deep autoencoder (DA), recurrent neural network (RNN), deep belief network (DBN), deep neural network (DNN), and deep conventional extreme machine learning (DC-EML). For research related to image processing, CNN got a lot of interest and was explored by the researcher. Various types of CNN architectures exist such as Alexnet [77], LeNet [78], Faster R-CNN [79], GoogLeNet [80], ResNet [81], etc. Basic information on various deep learning algorithms with its advantages and disadvantages are mentioned in Table 3.2.

Table 3.2 Basic information on various deep learning algorithms

Sr. no.	Deep learning algorithm	Basic information of algorithm	Advantages	Disadvantages
1.	Deep neural network (DNN)	It is a simple deep learning algorithm that has more than two hidden layers. Useful in applications related to classification and regression	Widely used with better performance and good accuracy	More time is required for the training process
2.	Convolution neural network (CNN)	It is a very good algorithm for image-related applications	The learning process of the network is fast and has good accuracy and performance	A lot of training labels are required for data in classification-related applications
3.	Recurrent neural network (RNN)	It is used as an algorithm of data in sequence format. The weights of the network are shared with all nodes of the network	Used in sequential operation-related application. Provides higher accuracy in applications related to recognition	Required big-size datasets for better performance
4.	Deep belief network (DBN)	It is useful in supervised learning as well as unsupervised learning. The hidden layer of each sub-network is available for the next sub-network	Greedy norms are used in each layer of the network to better predict the output	Required higher computational complexity in the training process
5.	Deep autoencoder (DA)	It is a supervised learning algorithm that is used for dimensional reduction of image features. The size of input and output is the same in this algorithm	Does not require labeled input data and different kinds of versions for a specific application such as de-noising autoencoder and sparse autoencoder. Provides more robustness to input data	Required pre-training process before using it
6.	Deep Boltzmann machine (DBM)	It is based on the properties of Boltzmann family. It is one of the extensions of RNN	More robust against interference and works effectively for discrete predicted value	For big dataset, optimization, utilization, and analysis of parameters are not possible

References

1. Bishop, C. (2006). *Pattern recognition and machine learning*. Berlin, Germany: Springer.
2. Murphy, K. (2012). *Machine learning – A probabilistic perspective*. Cambridge, MA: MIT Press.
3. Goodfellow, I., Bengio, Y., Courville, A., & Bengio, Y. (2016). *Deep learning* (Vol. 1). Cambridge, MA: MIT Press.

4. Kotsiantis, S. B. (2007). Supervised machine learning: A review of classification techniques. *Informatica, 31*, 249–268.
5. Thanki, R., & Borra, S. (2019). Application of machine learning algorithms for classification and security of diagnostic images. In *Machine learning in bio-signal analysis and diagnostic imaging* (pp. 273–292). London: Academic.
6. Borra, S., Thanki, R., & Dey, N. (2019). *Satellite image analysis: Clustering and classification*. Berlin, Germany: Springer.
7. Nath, S. S., Mishra, G., Kar, J., Chakraborty, S., & Dey, N. (2014, July). A survey of image classification methods and techniques. In *2014 international conference on Control, Instrumentation, Communication and Computational Technologies (ICCICCT)* (pp. 554–557). IEEE.
8. Jawak, S. D., Devliyal, P., & Luis, A. J. (2015). A comprehensive review on pixel oriented and object-oriented methods for information extraction from remotely sensed satellite images with a special emphasis on cryospheric applications. *Advances in Remote Sensing, 4*(03), 177.
9. Lillesand, T., Kiefer, R. W., & Chipman, J. (2014). *Remote sensing and image interpretation*. Hoboken, NJ: Wiley.
10. Zhang, H. (2004). The optimality of Naive Bayes. *AA, 1*(2), 3.
11. Schütze, H., Manning, C. D., & Raghavan, P. (2008). *Introduction to information retrieval* (Vol. 39). Cambridge, UK: Cambridge University Press.
12. McCallum, A., & Nigam, K. (1998, July). A comparison of event models for Naive Bayes text classification. In *AAAI-98 workshop on learning for text categorization* (Vol. 752, No. 1) (pp. 41–48).
13. Metsis, V., Androutsopoulos, I., & Paliouras, G. (2006, July). Spam filtering with naive Bayes-which naive Bayes? *CEAS, 17*, 28–69.
14. Yen, S. H., & Wang, C. J. (2006). SVM based watermarking technique. *Tamkang Journal of Science and Engineering, 9*(2), 141–150.
15. Vapnik, V. (1995). *The nature of statistical learning theory*. New York: Springer.
16. Hsu, C. W., Chang, C. C., & Lin, C. J. (2016). *A practical guide to support vector classification*. https://www.csie.ntu.edu.tw/~cjlin/papers/guide/guide.pdf. Last Access: February 2018.
17. Fisher, R. A. (1936). The use of multiple measurements in taxonomic problems. *Annals of Eugenics, 7*(2), 179–188.
18. Rao, C. R. (1948). The utilization of multiple measurements in problems of biological classification. *Journal of the Royal Statistical Society. Series B (Methodological), 10*(2), 159–203.
19. Mika, S., Ratsch, G., Weston, J., Scholkopf, B., & Mullers, K. R. (1999, August). Fisher discriminant analysis with kernels. In *Neural networks for signal processing IX, 1999. Proceedings of the 1999 IEEE Signal Processing Society workshop* (pp. 41–48). IEEE.
20. Friedman, J. H. (1989). Regularized discriminant analysis. *Journal of the American Statistical Association, 84*(405), 165–175.
21. Raschka, S. (2014). *Linear discriminant analysis*. Web link: https://sebastianraschka.com/Articles/2014_python_lda.html. Last Access: August 2018.
22. Saxena, R. (2017). *How decision tree algorithm works*. Web link: https://dataaspirant.com/2017/01/30/how-decision-tree-algorithm-works/. Last Access: August 2018.
23. Kulkarni, A. D., & Shrestha, A. (2017). Multispectral image analysis using decision trees. *International Journal of Advanced Computer Science and Applications, 8*(6), 11–18.
24. Quinlan, J. R. (1986). Induction of decision trees. *Machine Learning, 1*(1), 81–106.
25. Liaw, A., & Wiener, M. (2002). Classification and regression by random forest. *R News, 2*(3), 18–22.
26. Segal, M. R. (2004). *Machine learning benchmarks and random forest regression*. Dordrecht, The Netherlands: Kluwer Academic Publishers.
27. Cootes, T. F., Ionita, M. C., Lindner, C., & Sauer, P. (2012, October). Robust and accurate shape model fitting using random forest regression voting. In *European conference on Computer Vision* (pp. 278–291). Berlin, Heidelberg, Germany: Springer.

28. Synced. (2017). *How random forest algorithm works in machine learning*. Web link: https://syncedreview.com/2017/10/24/how-random-forest-algorithm-works-in-machine-learning/. Last Access: August 2018.
29. Polamuri, S. (2017). *How the random forest algorithm works in machine learning?* Web link: http://dataaspirant.com/2017/05/22/random-forest-algorithm-machine-learing/. Last Access: August 2018.
30. Kumar, D. N. (2014). *Remote sensing*. https://nptel.ac.in/courses/105108077/. Last Access: July 2018.
31. Wagstaff, K., Cardie, C., Rogers, S., & Schrödl, S. (2001, June). Constrained k-means clustering with background knowledge. *ICML, 1*, 577–584.
32. Hartigan, J. A., & Wong, M. A. (1979). Algorithm AS 136: A k-means clustering algorithm. *Journal of the Royal Statistical Society. Series C (Applied Statistics), 28*(1), 100–108.
33. Kanungo, T., Mount, D. M., Netanyahu, N. S., Piatko, C. D., Silverman, R., & Wu, A. Y. (2002). An efficient k-means clustering algorithm: Analysis and implementation. *IEEE Transactions on Pattern Analysis & Machine Intelligence, 7*, 881–892.
34. Alsabti, K., Ranka, S., & Singh, V. (1997). *An efficient k-means clustering algorithm*.
35. Likas, A., Vlassis, N., & Verbeek, J. J. (2003). The global k-means clustering algorithm. *Pattern Recognition, 36*(2), 451–461.
36. Kaufman, L., & Rousseeuw, P. J. (2009). *Finding groups in data: An introduction to cluster analysis* (Vol. 344). Hoboken, NJ: Wiley.
37. Jain, A. K., & Dubes, R. C. (1988). *Algorithms for clustering data*.
38. Mehrotra, K., Mohan, C. K., & Ranka, S. (1997). *Elements of artificial neural networks*. Cambridge, MA: MIT Press.
39. Jolliffe, I. (2011). Principal component analysis. In *International encyclopedia of statistical science* (pp. 1094–1096). Berlin, Heidelberg, Germany: Springer.
40. Abdi, H., & Williams, L. J. (2010). Principal component analysis. *Wiley Interdisciplinary Reviews: Computational Statistics, 2*(4), 433–459.
41. Celik, T. (2009). Unsupervised change detection in satellite images using principal component analysis and k-means clustering. *IEEE Geoscience and Remote Sensing Letters, 6*(4), 772–776.
42. Wold, S., Esbensen, K., & Geladi, P. (1987). Principal component analysis. *Chemometrics and Intelligent Laboratory Systems, 2*(1-3), 37–52.
43. Kwarteng, P., & Chavez, A. (1989). Extracting spectral contrast in Landsat Thematic Mapper image data using selective principal component analysis. *Photogrammetric Engineering and Remote Sensing, 55*, 339–348.
44. Rodarmel, C., & Shan, J. (2002). Principal component analysis for hyperspectral image classification. *Surveying and Land Information Science, 62*(2), 115–122.
45. Schowengerdt, R. A. (2006). *Remote sensing: Models and methods for image processing*. Saint Louis, MO: Elsevier.
46. Gonzalez, R. C., Woods, R. E., & Eddins, S. L. (2004). *Digital image processing using MATLAB* (Vol. 624). Upper Saddle River, NJ: Pearson-Prentice-Hall.
47. Fauvel, M., Chanussot, J., & Benediktsson, J. A. (2009). Kernel principal component analysis for the classification of hyperspectral remote sensing data over urban areas. *EURASIP Journal on Advances in Signal Processing, 2009*(1), 783194.
48. Dev, S., Wen, B., Lee, Y. H., & Winkler, S. (2016). Machine learning techniques and applications for ground-based image analysis. *arXiv preprint arXiv:1606.02811*.
49. Comon, P. (1994). Independent component analysis, a new concept? *Signal Processing, 36*(3), 287–314.
50. Xiao Benlin, A., Li Fangfang, B., Mao Xingliang, C., & Jin Huazhong, B. (2008). *Study on independent component analysis' application in classification and change detection of multispectral images*.
51. Dópido, I., Villa, A., Plaza, A., & Gamba, P. (2012). A quantitative and comparative assessment of unmixing-based feature extraction techniques for hyperspectral image classification.

IEEE Journal of Selected Topics in Applied Earth Observations and Remote Sensing, 5(2), 421–435.
52. Al-Taei, M. S. M., & Al-Ghrairi, A. H. T. (2016). Satellite image classification using moment and SVD method. *International Journal of Computer (IJC), 23*(1), 10–34.
53. Brindha, S. (2015). Satellite image enhancement using dwt–svd and segmentation using mrr–mrf model. *Journal of Network Communications and Emerging Technologies (JNCET), 1*(1).
54. Ranjith, K. J., Thomas, H. A., & Stamp, M. (2014). Singular value decomposition and metamorphic detection. *Journal of Computer Virology and Hacking Techniques, 11*(4), 203–216.
55. Biernacki, C., Celeux, G., & Govaert, G. (2000). Assessing a mixture model for clustering with the integrated completed likelihood. *IEEE Transactions on Pattern Analysis and Machine Intelligence, 22*(7), 719–725.
56. Biernacki, C., Celeux, G., & Govaert, G. (2003). Choosing starting values for the EM algorithm for getting the highest likelihood in multivariate Gaussian mixture models. *Computational Statistics & Data Analysis, 41*(3–4), 561–575.
57. Zivkovic, Z. (2004, August). Improved adaptive Gaussian mixture model for background subtraction. In *Proceedings of the 17th international conference on Pattern Recognition, 2004. ICPR 2004* (Vol. 2, pp. 28–31). IEEE.
58. Maugis, C., Celeux, G., & Martin-Magniette, M. L. (2009). Variable selection for clustering with Gaussian mixture models. *Biometrics, 65*(3), 701–709.
59. McLachlan, G., & Peel, D. (2000). *Finite mixture models* (Willey Series in Probability and Statistics). New York: Wiley.
60. Kohonen, T. (1982). Self-organized formation of topologically correct feature maps. *Biological Cybernetics, 43*(1), 59–69.
61. Kohonen, T. (1982). Analysis of a simple self-organizing process. *Biological Cybernetics, 44*(2), 135–140.
62. Ritter, H., & Kohonen, T. (1989). Self-organizing semantic maps. *Biological Cybernetics, 61*(4), 241–254.
63. Kangas, J. A., Kohonen, T. K., & Laaksonen, J. T. (1990). Variants of self-organizing maps. *IEEE Transactions on Neural Networks, 1*(1), 93–99.
64. Erwin, E., Obermayer, K., & Schulten, K. (1992). Self-organizing maps: Ordering, convergence properties and energy functions. *Biological Cybernetics, 67*(1), 47–55.
65. Kaski, S., Honkela, T., Lagus, K., & Kohonen, T. (1998). WEBSOM–Self-organizing maps of document collections. *Neurocomputing, 21*(1–3), 101–117.
66. Dittenbach, M., Merkl, D., & Rauber, A. (2000). The growing hierarchical self-organizing map. In *Proceedings of the IEEE-INNS-ENNS international joint conference on Neural Networks, 2000. IJCNN 2000* (Vol. 6, pp. 15–19). IEEE.
67. Fumo, D. (2017). *Types of machine learning algorithms you should know*. Web link: https://towardsdatascience.com/types-of-machine-learning-algorithms-you-should-know-953a08248861. Last Access: March 2020.
68. Q-learning in python. Web link: https://www.geeksforgeeks.org/q-learning-in-python/. Last Access: March 2020.
69. Moni, R. (SmartLab AI). (2019). *Reinforcement learning algorithms – An intuitive overview*. Web link: https://medium.com/@SmartLabAI/reinforcement-learning-algorithms-an-intuitive-overview-904e2dff5bbc
70. Reinforcement Learning Illustration. Web link: https://i.stack.imgur.com/eoeSq.png. Last Access: March 2020.
71. A basic introduction to neural networks. Website: http://pages.cs.wisc.edu/~bolo/shipyard/neural/local.html. Last Access: February 2018.
72. Caudill, M. (1989, February). Neural network primer: Part I. *AI Expert*.
73. Krizhevsky, A., Sutskever, I., & Hinton, G. E. (2012). ImageNet classification with deep convolutional neural networks. *Advances in Neural Information Processing Systems*, 1097–1105.
74. Lawrence, S., Giles, C. L., Tsoi, A. C., & Back, A. D. (1997). Face recognition: A convolutional neural-network approach. *IEEE Transactions on Neural Networks, 8*(1), 98–113.

75. Kandi, H., Mishra, D., & Gorthi, S. R. S. (2017). Exploring the learning capabilities of convolutional neural networks for robust image watermarking. *Computers & Security, 65*, 247–268.
76. Mun, S. M., Nam, S. H., Jang, H. U., Kim, D., & Lee, H. K. (2017). A robust blind watermarking using convolutional neural network. *ArXiv preprint arXiv: 1704.03248*.
77. Alexnet. Web link: https://github.com/BVLC/caffe/tree/master/models/bvlc_alexnet. Last access: February 2019.
78. LeNet. Web link: http://deeplearning.net/tutorial/lenet.html. Last access: February 2019.
79. Faster R-CNN. Web link: https://github.com/rbgirshick/py-faster-rcnn. Last access: February 2019.
80. GoogLeNet. Web link: https://leonardoaraujosantos.gitbooks.io/artificial-inteligence/content/googlenet.html. Last access: February 2019.
81. ResNet. Web link: https://github.com/gcr/torch-residual-networks. Last access: February 2019.

Chapter 4
AI in Healthcare and Medical Imaging

In Chap. 3, we learned information regarding artificial intelligence and various learning algorithms. In this chapter, we will discuss the role of artificial intelligence in healthcare and medical imaging and its several tools and technologies available in the market.

4.1 AI in Healthcare

AI in healthcare is used to interpret, analyze, and visualize complex medical data using various algorithms. AI is the ability to make a conclusive decision based on the given input data without interference of human input. AI technology differs from the conventional technologies used in healthcare where data is collected and processed and provides a better decision to the end-user. AI technology uses various machine learning algorithms and deep learning algorithms that can analyze medical data patterns and create their own decision. For a better conclusive decision, AI algorithms need to be simulated and tested repeatedly. These algorithms behave differently from humans in two ways: (1) algorithms are written in such a way that it cannot adjust itself as per the input data and can only perform a predefined task, and (2) some algorithms have hidden layers that give prefer decision and prediction but not the cause or the why [1].

The main aim of AI-based healthcare applications is to analyze relationships between diagnosis and treatment method and conclusive decision [2]. AI technologies are being developed and applied to practice in various areas of healthcare as a diagnostic method, treatment protocol development, medicine or drug development, health monitoring, etc. Recently, many medical institutions around the world developed AI-based algorithms for various applications in healthcare. Companies like IBM, Google, and Intel also developed various AI-based applications for healthcare [3, 4]. Additionally, hospitals are looking

K. Shaikh et al., *Artificial Intelligence in Breast Cancer Early Detection and Diagnosis*, https://doi.org/10.1007/978-3-030-59208-0_4

for AI software to support operational initiatives that increase cost-saving, improve patient satisfaction, and meet their staffing and workforce needs [5]. Many companies and startups are developing predictive analytics solutions that help healthcare managers improve business operations through increasing utilization, decreasing patient boarding, reducing the length of stay, and optimizing staffing levels [6].

The system based on AI was developed in the early 1970s which was known as Dendral [7]. This system was designed for applications in organic chemistry which provided the basis for a subsequent system MYCIN [8]. This is the first application of AI in the development of medicine [9, 10]. Around the 1980s and the early 1990s, the advancement in computer algorithms and networking helped researchers and developers to believe in AI systems and paved the way for these systems of healthcare to be designed which perform better in the absence of perfect data and provide a conclusive decision to doctors [11]. These systems are used in various learning approaches such as fuzzy set theory, Bayesian networks, and artificial neural networks to achieve an intelligent solution for healthcare data [12]. Advancements in various technologies have enabled the growth of healthcare-related applications of AI [13–18]:

- Faster collection and processing of data
- Development of various types of databases
- Proper designing of a system for electronic health records
- Improved human perceptual and decision abilities
- Development of robotics-based treatment methods

4.1.1 AI-Based Healthcare Research

In the last 10 years, research and development are conducted in AI-based systems within various areas of healthcare. These areas are radiology, medical imaging, healthcare monitoring systems, drug development, etc.

- *Radiology*: AI-based system detects minor changes in medical images that can be accidentally missed by the lab radiologist. One example is the AI-based algorithm for pneumonia detection developed by the research team from Stanford University which gives better results compared to radiologist prediction [19]. Recently, many companies provide different AI-based platforms where medical images can be uploaded, and the decision outcome is based on an input image. These platforms are developed with the help of various AI-based algorithms such as machine learning and deep learning.
- *Imaging*: A lot of research is advancing on the development of various AI-based systems with the help of medical images. These systems detect various types of

diseases such as cancer, diabetes, glaucoma, etc. based on input types of medical images.

- *Disease diagnosis*: Many diseases can be efficiently and accurately diagnosed with the help of AI-based systems. Some of the diseases such as cancer, diabetes, and cardiovascular have had accurate diagnoses with the help of AI-based system, a product of several research and testing [20]. In 2017, Jiang et al. [21] give a review of various AI-based systems for different types of disease diagnosis. These systems use various algorithms such as SVM, neural networks, decision trees, and many more.
- *Telehealth*: The development of an AI-based system arises with the readily increasing usage of telemedicine [22]. The ability of the system to monitor the health of patients using AI allows the transfer of important health information to doctors for better diagnosis and treatment of disease [22].
- *Drug development and interactions*: Various drug development algorithms are available in the literature which show significant use of AI [23]. The OCD (obsessive-compulsive disorder) drug molecule DSP-1181 was invented and developed by Exscientia (British startup) and Sumitomo Dainippon Pharma (Japanese pharmaceutical firm) [23]. Due to the improvement in natural language processing (NLP), many new algorithms were developed by researchers for study about the effects of drugs on human body [24–27]. Drug interactions provide a threat risk for patients taking multiple medications simultaneously.

4.1.2 Application of AI in Healthcare

Many industries have been hit by the advent of new technologies in the information age. According to a 2016 report from CB Insights, 86% of healthcare providers, life science companies, and healthcare technology vendors use artificial intelligence technology. By 2020, these companies will spend an average of US$ 54 million on artificial intelligence projects. The following are the common applications of AI which are changing the recent healthcare industry and in the future [28].

- *Maintaining healthcare data*: Since the first step in healthcare is compiling and analyzing information (such as medical records and other histories), data management is a widely used application of artificial intelligence and digital automation. AI-based systems collect, store, reformat, and trace data to provide faster and more consistent access.
- *Doing repetitive jobs*: AI-based systems can perform tests, x-rays, CT scans, data entry, and other mundane tasks faster and more accurately. Cardiology and radiology are two disciplines where the amount of data is huge to analyze and time-consuming. Future cardiologists and radiologists should look only at the most critical cases in which human monitoring is useful.

- *Design of treatment method*: Artificial intelligence systems are created to analyze data—notes and reports—from a patient's file, external research, and clinical expertise to help you choose the right, individually customized treatment pathway.
- *Digital consultation*: Apps like Babylon in the United Kingdom use AI to provide medical consultation based on personal medical history and general medical knowledge. Users report their symptoms to the app, which uses speech recognition to compare it with a database of illnesses. Considering the user's medical history, Babylon offers recommended action.
- *Virtual nurses*: There are startups which has developed digital nurse, who helps people monitor the condition of patients and follow treatments between doctor visits. This program uses machine learning to support patients, specializing in chronic illnesses. In 2016, Boston Children's Hospital developed an app for Amazon Alexa that provides basic health information and advice to parents of sick children. The app answers to questions about symptoms and whether a visit to the doctor is needed.
- *Medication management*: The Patient Institute of Health has developed a unique app to monitor the use of a patient's medication, with the use of a smartphone's webcam partnered with AI to automatically verify that patients are taking their prescriptions and help them manage their condition. Most common users are people with serious medical conditions, patients who go against doctors' advice, and those who participate in clinical trials.
- *Drug creation*: It takes more than a decade and billions of dollars to develop CE actions through clinical trials. Making this process faster and cheaper can change the world. Amid the recent Ebola virus threat, an AI-powered program has been used to scan existing drugs that can be re-designed to fight the disease. This type of analysis usually finds two actions that reduce the risk of Ebola infection in one day, and this type of analysis usually takes months or years a difference that can save thousands of lives.
- *Precision medicine*: Genetics and its look for mutations and links to disease from information in DNA. With the help of AI, body scans can detect cancer and vascular diseases in advance and predict the health risks people will face based on their genetics.
- *Health monitoring*: Wearable health trackers like Fitbit, Apple, Garmin, and others monitor heart rate and activity levels. They can send alerts to the user to get more exercise and share this information with physicians (and AI systems) for additional data points on patients' needs and habits.
- *Healthcare system analysis*: In the Netherlands, 97% of healthcare invoices are digital. A Dutch company uses AI to shift data and help healthcare systems avoid unnecessary patient hospitalization to highlight inefficiencies in treatment and workflow.

4.1.3 Industries Work in Healthcare Area

The subsequent motive of large health companies merging with other health companies allows for greater health data accessibility [29]. Greater health data may allow for more implementation of AI algorithms [30]. A large part of the industry which focuses on implementation of AI in the healthcare sector is the clinical decision support systems [31]. As the number of data increases, AI decision support systems become more efficient. Numerous companies are exploring the possibilities of the incorporation of big data in the healthcare industry [32].

The following are examples of large companies that have contributed to AI algorithms for use in healthcare.

- *IBM*: IBM's Watson Oncology is in development at Memorial Sloan Kettering Cancer Center and Cleveland Clinic [33]. IBM is also working with CVS Health on AI applications in chronic disease treatment and with Johnson & Johnson on the analysis of scientific papers to find new connections for drug development [34]. In May 2017, IBM and Rensselaer Polytechnic Institute began a joint project entitled Health Empowerment by Analytics, Learning, and Semantics (HEALS), to explore using AI technology to enhance healthcare [35].
- *Microsoft*: Microsoft's Project Hanover, in partnership with Oregon Health and Science University's Knight Cancer Institute, analyzes medical research to predict the most effective cancer drug treatment options for patients [36]. Other projects include medical image analysis of tumor progression and the development of programmable cells [37].
- *Google*: Google's DeepMind platform is being used by the UK National Health Service to detect certain health risks through data collected via a mobile app [38]. A second project with the NHS involves an analysis of medical images collected from NHS patients to develop computer vision algorithms to detect cancerous tissues [39].
- *Intel*: Intel's venture capital arm Intel Capital recently invested with the startup Lumiata which uses AI to identify risk patients and develop care options [40].
- Others: Digital consultant apps like Babylon Health's GP at Hand, Ada Health, and Your.MD use AI to give medical consultation [41] based on personal medical history and common medical knowledge. Users report their symptoms into the app, which uses speech recognition to compare against a database of illnesses. Babylon then offers a recommended action, taking into account the user's medical history. Entrepreneurs in healthcare have been effectively using seven business model archetypes to take AI solutions to the marketplace. These archetypes depend on the value generated for the target user (e.g., patient focus vs. healthcare provider and payer focus) and value capturing mechanisms (e.g., providing information or connecting stakeholders) [42].

4.2 AI in Medical Imaging

Doctors have been using medical imaging techniques to diagnose diseases like cancer for many years. However, artificial intelligence (AI) has the potential to take this technology further and to improve medical imaging capabilities such as higher automation and increased productivity. AI can improve medical imaging processes like image analysis and help with patient diagnosis. With many applied AI solutions and many more AI applications showing promising scientific test results, the market for AI in medical imaging is forecast to grow exponentially over the next few years.

Medical imaging uses different processes and imaging methods to represent an internal image of the human body for diagnostic and treatment purposes. Medical imaging is often used in treatment and follow-ups for diagnosed diseases. The term medical imaging includes various radiological imaging techniques such as x-ray radiography, magnetic resonance imaging (MRI), medical ultrasonography or ultrasound, and computed tomography (CT) and nuclear medicine functional imaging techniques like positron emission tomography (PET). AI can improve traditional medical imaging methods like computed tomography (CT), magnetic resonance imaging (MRI), and x-ray by offering computational capabilities that process images with greater speed and accuracy at scale. AI has the potential to improve medical imaging with:

- *Higher automation*: AI can automate parts of the radiology workflow.
- *Increased productivity*: AI has better computational capabilities than humans, so it can analyze medical images faster than medical doctors.
- *Standardized processes*: AI can supply doctors with AI tools to compute big data and help and encourage doctors to work smarter and more efficiently.
- *More accurate diagnosis*: Studies show that AI can be more efficient than doctors and experts at diagnosing many diseases like cancer from medical images. For example, scientists at Google have created an AI that diagnoses breast cancer. The AI is fed with slides of medical images and uses DL algorithms to diagnose cancerous cells. The AI recorded a 99% accuracy in cancer diagnosis based on these slides compared to 38% of some doctors in the comparison group.
- *Computing quantitative data*: AI can use quantitative data in ways that are beyond the limits of human cognition. For example, AI can predict if a patient will suffer from heart failure based on their medical history and rate of hospital visits.
- *Assistance for doctors*: AI can compute a large amount of data, map it, and represent the relevant parts in a brief and efficient format that doctors can use.

4.2.1 Various Types of Medical Imaging Techniques

In this section, various types of medical imaging techniques are described. There are mainly four types of medical imaging techniques: x-ray, MRI, CT, and US. The details of these techniques are given below:

- *x-ray imaging*: The first medical imaging technique is invented by Hall-Edwards for the observation of internal organs of human bodies. This technique is known as x-ray imaging. Here, x-rays are passed through disease-affected organs of the patient's body, and the result is acquired on the x-ray film. The images generated using these imaging techniques are less expensive and easy to be carried from one place to another. But the image generated using this technique has low quality, and sometimes, it is difficult to get information from it.
- *Ultrasonography (US) imaging*: The second major medical imaging technique is invented by I. Edler and C. Hertz in 1953. This technique is known as ultrasonography (US) imaging. In this technique, the ultrasonic signals are passed through the human skin by a transducer, and the same transducer receives echoes that are generated due to impedance differences in the tissue of a human. These echoes are amplified, processed, and displayed on the monitor as digital signals. Dr. Rao [43] has beautifully explained how this imaging technique works. US images have low perceptual quality and are difficult to interpret.
- *Computed tomography (CT) imaging*: The third major medical imaging technique is invented by A. Cormack and G. Hounsfield in 1972. This technique is known as computed tomography or computer tomography (CT). This image is generated by passing x-rays in multiple directions through disease-affected organs of the patient's body. Recently, images generated using this technique are widely used in the treatment of health problems related to neurology, cardiology, and gastroenterology.
- *Magnetic resonance imaging (MRI)*: The fourth major medical imaging technique is invented by P. Lauterbur and P. Mansfield in 1973. This technique is known as magnetic resonance imaging (MRI). In this technique, the helium liquid-cooled magnetic field is used for the generation of the image. This imaging technique generates a 3D medical image and is widely used in health problems related to neurology, gastroenterology, and angiography.

Recently some new medical imaging techniques arrived in the market due to enhancements in basic sciences such as nuclear and lighting. This technique is known as positron emission tomography (PET) and endoscopy. These techniques are used for better diagnosis and treatment of the patient. PET images are used for the diagnosis of different types of tumor detection and treatments related to cancer. Endoscopy is invented around 2001 and is used to get optical images of the internal body. In 2010, General Electric (GE) introduced new medical image techniques by a combination of CT and MR images with PET images for better health-related treatment.

4.2.2 Computer-Aided Detection (CADe) and Computer-Aided Diagnosis (CADx)

Computer-aided detection (CADe) and computer-aided diagnosis (CADx) are systems that help doctors in understanding medical images. Various imaging techniques such as x-ray, MRI, and CT have numerous amount of information which doctors or other medical professionals have to analyze and evaluate perfectly within a short period. These systems process digital images in various approaches and give important information within the images that help for better detection and prediction of disease within it. These systems are interdisciplinary technologies, which combine various technologies such as artificial intelligence and computer vision for better analysis of medical images. CADe systems usually detect conspicuous structures, while the CADx system evaluates these structures. For the last 50 years, this system had been used in clinical environments. This system does not provide a complete solution but plays supporting roles. The doctor is finally responsible for the interpretation of a medical image. However, the goal of CAD systems is to detect the earliest signs of abnormality in patients that doctors cannot such as tumors of cancer, glaucoma, etc. [44, 45].

Around 1950, researchers in various fields of computers started exploring the possibility of the development of a computer-aided system for diagnosis and detection of disease with the help of medical images. The first CAD system was developed using various flow charts, pattern matching, and knowledge-based assumptions for better decision-making regarding prediction and diagnosis of disease [46]. Since the early 1970s, some CAD systems were developed and used for educational purposes. Some of the practical examples of CAD systems are MYCIA, INTERNIST-I expert system, and CADUCEUS [47–49].

4.2.2.1 The Methodology of the CAD System

The CAD system is fundamentally a computer vision-based complex system where the pattern in images is identified. Various types of medical images are used for the detection of suspicious structures in it. Normally, thousands of medical images are used to optimize the performance of the system. Digital medical image data are copied to a CAD server in DICOM format. Then data are prepared and analyzed in several steps. Generally, CAD systems involve various steps of preprocessing, segmentation, feature extraction, and classification, as shown in Fig. 4.1 [50].

- *Preprocessing*: This step of a CAD system improves the quality of the input medical image. It used various medical image algorithms such as noise removal, filtering, etc. to perform various operations such as reduction of artifacts, reduction of noise in an image, increasing contrast of an image, etc.
- *Segmentation*: Image segmentation plays a very significant role in the detection of suspicious regions that are used for further analysis. During this operation,

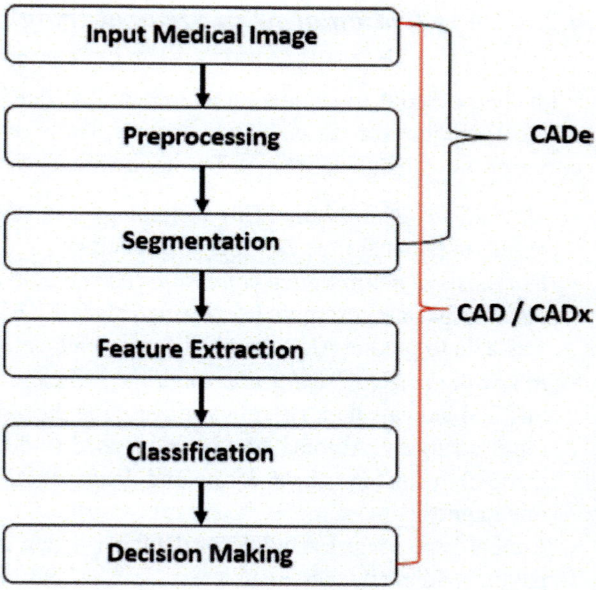

Fig. 4.1 General framework of CADe/CADx system

various information such as the differentiation of organs like heart, lung, blood vessels, etc., possible round lesions, and sample gray values in a volume of interest are extracted from the image [51].

- *Feature Extraction*: This is one of the important steps in the CAD system where a segmented structure or region of interest (ROI) is analyzed and important information is obtained from it, such as compactness, size, and location of the tumor, reference organ near close to ROIs, and average gray level value analysis within the ROI.
- *Classification*: After segmentation and feature extraction, the suspicious area can be categorized as normal or abnormal based on selected features using various classification techniques. Various classification algorithms such as k-nearest neighbors, naïve Bayesian classifier, support vector machine, artificial neural network, etc. are used for this purpose.

4.2.2.2 Evaluation of the CAD System

The performance of the CAD system is measured by two major factors such as sensitivity and specificity, and they seek for suspicious structure. CAD systems may not perform 100%, but their hit rate means sensitivity can be up to 98% in present scenarios. However, the accuracy of the CAD depends on conditions of the medical images used for training of the system and various selected features such as quality of images, radiologist's marks, tumor size and location, etc. The selection of features may have influences in the performance of the CAD system.

4.2.3 Application of AI in Medical Imaging

With the potential to improve and standardize the process, AI can be applied in medical imaging for various medical tasks. However, AI is intended to be used in conjunction with human insight. The applications of AI in medical imaging include:

- *Medical image analysis*: This technology can identify anomalies and diseases based on medical images better than doctors.
- *Diagnosis of neurological conditions*: AI can help doctors diagnose neurological diseases like amyotrophic lateral sclerosis (ALS). A study has also shown that AI was able to predict Alzheimer's disease years before it manifests.
- *Revealing cardiovascular abnormalities*: AI can measure a patient's heart structure and indicate their risk of cardiovascular disease or other problems that might require surgery. Automated AI can be used to detect abnormalities in common medical tests like chest x-ray and lead to quicker risk detection and less misdiagnosis.
- *Cancer screening*: Early cancer diagnosis often results in a better outcome for patients. Recently, scientists created an AI based on convolutional neural networks (CNN), a type of artificial neural network (ANN) used to identify various types of cancer with a high success rate. These experiments show that AI can decrease detection times and improve the rate of diagnosis.

References

1. Algorithms Need Managers, Too. *Harvard Business Review* (2016). Weblink: https://hbr.org/2016/01/algorithms-need-managers-too. Last Access: April 2020.
2. Coiera, E. (1997). *Guide to medical informatics, the internet and telemedicine*. London: Chapman & Hall, Ltd.
3. Power, B. (2015). *Artificial intelligence is almost ready for business*. Massachusetts General Hospital. Weblink: https://hbr.org/2015/03/artificial-intelligence-is-almost-ready-for-business. Last Access: April 2020
4. Bloch-Budzier, S. (2016). *NHS using Google technology to treat patients*. Weblink: https://www.bbc.com/news/health-38055509. Last Access: April 2020.
5. Lorenzetti, L. (2016). *Here is how IBM Watson Health is transforming the health care industry*. Weblink: http://fortune.com/ibm-watson-health-business-strategy/. Last Access: April 2020.
6. HealthIT Analytics. (2018). *Providers embrace predictive analytics for clinical, financial benefits*. Weblink: https://healthitanalytics.com/news/providers-embrace-predictive-analytics-for-clinical-financial-benefits. Last Access: April 2020.
7. Lindsay, R. K., Buchanan, B. G., Feigenbaum, E. A., & Lederberg, J. (1993). DENDRAL: A case study of the first expert system for scientific hypothesis formation. *Artificial Intelligence, 61*(2), 209–261.
8. Clancey, W. J., & Shortliffe, E. H. (Eds.). (1984). *Readings in medical artificial intelligence. The first decade*. Reading, MA: Addison-Wesley Longman Publishing Co., Inc.
9. Shortliffe, E. H., & Buchanan, B. G. (Eds.). (1985). *Rule-based expert systems: The MYCIN experiments of the Stanford heuristic programming project*. Reading, MA: Addison-Wesley Publishing Company.

10. Duda, R. O., & Shortliffe, E. H. (1983). Expert systems research. *Science, 220*(4594), 261–268.
11. Miller, R. A. (1994). Medical diagnostic decision support systems—past, present, and future: A threaded bibliography and brief commentary. *Journal of the American Medical Informatics Association, 1*(1), 8–27.
12. Adlassnig, K. P. (1980). A fuzzy logical model of computer-assisted medical diagnosis. *Methods of Information in Medicine, 19*(03), 141–148.
13. Koomey, J., Berard, S., Sanchez, M., & Wong, H. (2010). Implications of historical trends in the electrical efficiency of computing. *IEEE Annals of the History of Computing, 33*(3), 46–54.
14. Barnes, B., & Dupré, J. (2009). *Genomes and what to make of them*. Chicago: University of Chicago Press.
15. Jha, A. K., DesRoches, C. M., Campbell, E. G., Donelan, K., Rao, S. R., Ferris, T. G., et al. (2009). Use of electronic health records in US hospitals. *New England Journal of Medicine, 360*(16), 1628–1638.
16. Banko, M., & Brill, E. (2001, July). Scaling to very very large corpora for natural language disambiguation. In *Proceedings of the 39th annual meeting on Association for Computational Linguistics* (pp. 26–33). Association for Computational Linguistics.
17. Dougherty, G. (2009). *Digital image processing for medical applications*. Cambridge, UK: Cambridge University Press.
18. Artificial Intelligence and Machine Learning for Healthcare. *Sigmoidal* (2017). Weblink: https://sigmoidal.io/artificial-intelligence-and-machine-learning-for-healthcare/. Last Access: April 2020.
19. Rajpurkar, P., Irvin, J., Zhu, K., Yang, B., Mehta, H., Duan, T., & Lungren, M. P. (2017). Chexnet: Radiologist-level pneumonia detection on chest x-rays with deep learning. *ArXiv preprint arXiv*: 1711.05225.
20. Alić, B., Gurbeta, L., & Badnjević, A. (2017, June). Machine learning techniques for classification of diabetes and cardiovascular diseases. In *2017 Sixth Mediterranean conference on Embedded Computing (MECO)* (pp. 1–4). Piscataway, NJ: IEEE.
21. Jiang, F., Jiang, Y., Zhi, H., Dong, Y., Li, H., Ma, S., et al. (2017). Artificial intelligence in healthcare: Past, present and future. *Stroke and Vascular Neurology, 2*(4), 230–243.
22. Pacis, D. M. M., Subido, E. D., Jr., & Bugtai, N. T. (2018, February). Trends in telemedicine utilizing artificial intelligence. In *AIP conference proceedings* (Vol. 1933, No. 1, p. 040009). New York: AIP Publishing LLC.
23. Artificial intelligence created medicine to be used on humans for first time. *BBC News* (2020). Weblink: https://www.bbc.com/news/technology-51315462. Last Access: April 2020.
24. Bokharaeian, B., & Diaz, A. (2016). Extraction of drug-drug interaction from literature through detecting linguistic-based negation and clause dependency. *Journal of AI and Data Mining, 4*(2), 203–212.
25. Cai, R., Liu, M., Hu, Y., Melton, B. L., Matheny, M. E., Xu, H., et al. (2017). Identification of adverse drug-drug interactions through causal association rule discovery from spontaneous adverse event reports. *Artificial Intelligence in Medicine, 76*, 7–15.
26. Christopoulou, F., Tran, T. T., Sahu, S. K., Miwa, M., & Ananiadou, S. (2020). Adverse drug events and medication relation extraction in electronic health records with ensemble deep learning methods. *Journal of the American Medical Informatics Association, 27*(1), 39–46.
27. Zhou, D., Miao, L., & He, Y. (2018). Position-aware deep multi-task learning for drug–drug interaction extraction. *Artificial Intelligence in Medicine, 87*, 1–8.
28. Swetha. (2018). *10 common applications of artificial intelligence in healthcare*. Weblink: https://medium.com/artificial-intelligence-usm-systems/10-common-applications-of-artificial-intelligence-in-health-care-9d34ccccda5c. Last Access: April. 2020.
29. Monica, P. R. (2018). What merger mania means for health care. *CNNMoney*. Weblink: http://money.cnn.com/2018/03/08/investing/health-care-mergers-cigna-express-scripts-consolidation/index.html. Last Access: May 2020.
30. Leaf, C. (2018). Why you are the reason for those health care mergers. *Fortune*. Weblink: https://fortune.com/2018/03/19/cvs-aetna-healthcare-mergers-big-data/. Last Access: May 2020.

31. Horvitz, E. J., Breese, J. S., & Henrion, M. (1988). Decision theory in expert systems and artificial intelligence. *International Journal of Approximate Reasoning, 2*(3), 247–302.
32. Arnold, D., & Wilson, T. (2017). *What doctor? Why AI and robotics will define new health*. London: PwC.
33. Cohn, J. (2013). The robot will see you now. *The Atlantic*. Weblink: https://www.theatlantic.com/magazine/archive/2013/03/the-robot-will-see-you-now/309216/. Last Access: May 2020.
34. Lorenzetti, L. (2016). From cancer to consumer tech: A look inside IBM's Watson Health Strategy. *Fortune*. Weblink: http://fortune.com/ibm-watson-health-business-strategy/. Last Access: May 2020.
35. IBM and Rensselaer Team to Research Chronic Diseases with Cognitive Computing. (2017). Weblink: https://news.rpi.edu/content/2017/05/17/ibm-and-rensselaer-team-research-chronic-diseases-cognitive-computing. Last Access: May 2020.
36. Bass, D. (2016). Microsoft develops AI to help cancer doctors find the right treatments. *Bloomberg*. Weblink: https://www.bloomberg.com/news/articles/2016-09-20/microsoft-develops-ai-to-help-cancer-doctors-find-the-right-treatments. Last Access: May 2020.
37. Knapton, S. (2016). Microsoft will 'solve' cancer within 10 years by 'reprogramming' diseased cells. *The Telegraph*. Weblink: https://www.telegraph.co.uk/science/2016/09/20/microsoft-will-solve-cancer-within-10-years-by-reprogramming-dis/. Last Access: May 2020.
38. Bloch-Budzier, S. (2016). NHS teams with Google to treat patients. *BBC News*. Weblink: https://www.bbc.com/news/health-38055509. Last Access: May 2020.
39. Baraniuk, C. (2016). Google gets access to cancer scans. *BBC News*. Weblink: https://www.bbc.com/news/technology-37230806. Last Access: May 2020.
40. Primack, D. (2016). Intel capital cancels $1 billion portfolio sale. *Fortune*. Weblink: http://fortune.com/2016/05/26/intel-capital-cancels-1-billion-portfolio-sale/. Last Access: May 2020.
41. Parkin, S. (2016, 9 March). *The artificially intelligent doctor will hear you now*. MIT Technology. Weblink: https://www.technologyreview.com/s/600868/the-artificially-intelligent-doctor-will-hear-you-now/. Last Access: May 2020.
42. Garbuio, M., & Lin, N. (2019). Artificial intelligence as a growth engine for health care startups: Emerging business models. *California Management Review, 61*(2), 59–83.
43. Rao, K., & Rao, V. (2006). *Medical image processing*. In Proceedings of workshop on medical image processing and applications.
44. Bird, R. E., Wallace, T. W., & Yankaskas, B. C. (1992). Analysis of cancers missed at screening mammography. *Radiology, 184*(3), 613–617.
45. Baker, J. A., Rosen, E. L., Lo, J. Y., Gimenez, E. I., Walsh, R., & Soo, M. S. (2003). Computer-aided detection (CAD) in screening mammography: Sensitivity of commercial CAD systems for detecting architectural distortion. *American Journal of Roentgenology, 181*(4), 1083–1088.
46. Yanase, J., & Triantaphyllou, E. (2019). A systematic survey of computer-aided diagnosis in medicine: Past and present developments. *Expert Systems with Applications, 138*, 112821.
47. Shortliffe, E. H., & Buchanan, B. G. (1975). A model of inexact reasoning in medicine. *Mathematical Biosciences, 23*(3–4), 351–379.
48. Miller, R. A., Pople Jr., H. E., & Myers, J. D. (1982). Internist-I, an experimental computer-based diagnostic consultant for general internal medicine. *New England Journal of Medicine, 307*(8), 468–476.
49. Feigenbaum, E. A., & McCorduck, P. (1984). *The fifth generation* (p. 52). London: Pan Books.
50. Koundal, D., & Sharma, B. (2019). Advanced neutrosophic set-based ultrasound image analysis. In *Neutrosophic set in medical image analysis* (pp. 51–73). New York: Academic.
51. Echegaray, S., Gevaert, O., Shah, R., Kamaya, A., Louie, J., Kothary, N., et al. (2015). Core samples for radiomics features that are insensitive to tumor segmentation: Method and pilot study using CT images of hepatocellular carcinoma. *Journal of Medical Imaging, 2*(4), 041011.

Chapter 5
Breast Cancer Detection and Diagnosis Using AI

In the previous chapter, we discussed the role of AI in healthcare and medical imaging. In this chapter, we focus on various imaging techniques and stages for the detection and diagnosis of breast cancer with its benefits and risks.

5.1 Various Imaging Techniques for the Detection of Breast Cancer

The design and developments in the detection and diagnosis system of breast cancer had significantly improved in the last two decades. Various imaging tools such as mammography and ultrasound are widely used for the treatment of breast cancer. The screening of these images has contributed significantly to better detection and diagnosis of breast cancer. Nowadays, digital imaging technologies are used, which may aid with a computer-aided detection system for cancer. The advancement in ultrasound, MRI, and nuclear medicine also has been significantly used in the detection and diagnosis of breast cancer. The next subsections give information on various imaging technologies that are used for the treatment of breast cancer.

5.1.1 Breast Mammography

Two-dimensional x-ray images of the breasts have been used as a cancer screening tool for the last 30 years and are still being used nowadays in most hospitals to screen breast cancer. A mammogram is an x-ray of the breast that allows doctors to look for changes in breast tissue [1].

A mammogram can often find or detect breast cancer early when it is small, even before a lump can be felt. The mammogram can be divided into two types such as

K. Shaikh et al., *Artificial Intelligence in Breast Cancer Early Detection and Diagnosis*, https://doi.org/10.1007/978-3-030-59208-0_5

screening mammograms and diagnostic mammograms [2]. A screening mammogram is used to look for signs of breast cancer in women who do not have any breast symptoms or problems. X-ray pictures of each breast are taken, typically from two different angles. Mammograms can also be used to look at a woman's breast if she has breast symptoms or if a change is seen on a screening mammogram. When used in this way, they are called diagnostic mammograms. They may include extra views (images) of the breast that are not part of screening mammograms. Sometimes diagnostic mammograms are used to screen women who are treated for breast cancer in the past. Mammograms can often show abnormal areas in the breast. They cannot prove that an abnormal area is a cancer, but they can help healthcare providers decide whether more testing is needed.

A mammogram uses a machine designed to look only at a breast tissue. The machine takes x-rays at lower doses than usual x-rays. Because these x-rays do not go through tissue easily, the machine has two plates that compress or flatten the breast to spread the tissue apart. This gives a better picture and allows less radiation to be used. The doctor reading your mammogram will be looking for different types of breast changes, such as small white spots called calcifications, larger abnormal areas called masses, and other suspicious areas that could be signs of cancer [1–3]. A sample of a breast mammogram is shown in Fig. 5.1.

- *Calcifications:* Calcifications are tiny calcium deposits within the breast tissue. They look like small white spots on a mammogram. They may or may not be caused by cancer. There are two types of calcifications such as macrocalcifications and microcalcifications. Macrocalcifications are larger calcium deposits that are most likely due to changes caused by aging of the breast arteries, old injuries, or inflammation. These deposits are typically related to non-cancerous conditions and do not need to be checked for cancer with a biopsy. Macrocalcifications become more common as women get older (especially after age 50). Microcalcifications are tiny specks of calcium in the breast. When seen on a mammogram, they are more of a concern than macrocalcifications, but they do not always mean that cancer is present. The shape and layout of microcalcifications help the radiologist judge how likely it is that the change is due to cancer. In most cases, microcalcifications do not need to be checked with a biopsy. However, if they have a suspicious look and pattern, a biopsy will be recommended to check for cancer.
- *Masses:* A mass is an area of dense breast tissue with a shape and edges that make it look different from the rest of the breast tissue. With or without calcifications, it is another important change seen on a mammogram. Masses can be many things, including cysts (non-cancerous, fluid-filled sacs) and non-cancerous solid tumors (such as fibroadenomas), but they may also be a sign of cancer. Cysts are fluid-filled sacs. Simple cysts (fluid-filled sacs with thin walls) are not cancer and do not need to be checked with a biopsy. If a mass is not a simple cyst, it is of more concern, so a biopsy might be needed to be sure it is not cancer. Solid masses can be more concerning, but most breast masses are not cancer. A cyst and a solid mass can feel the same. They can also look the same on a

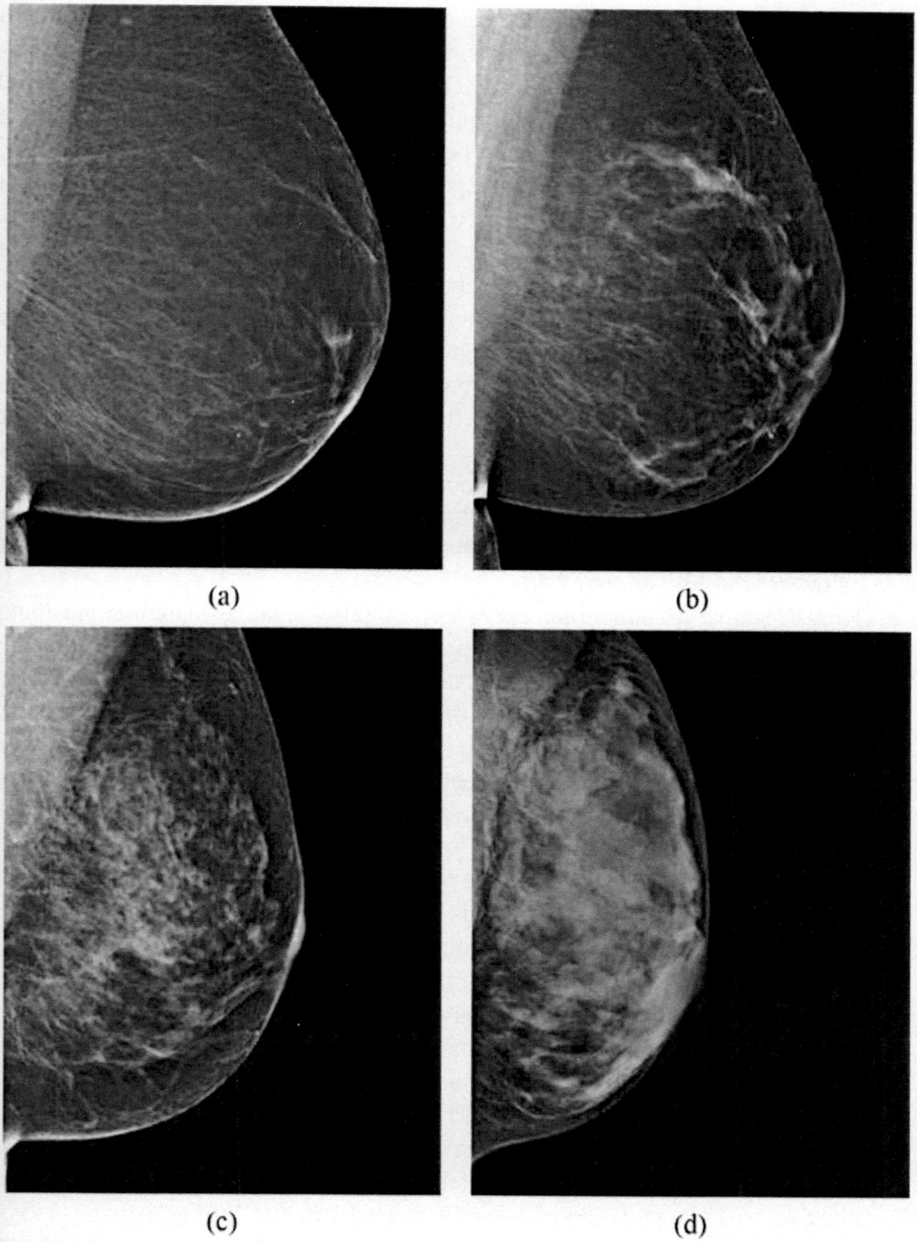

Fig. 5.1 Different types of breast mammograms: (**a**) all fatty tissues, (**b**) scattered areas of dense glandular and fibrous tissue, (**c**) dense glandular and fibrous tissue, (**d**) extremely dense tissue

mammogram. The doctor must be sure it is a cyst to know it is not cancer. To be sure, a breast ultrasound is often done because it is a better tool to see fluid-filled sacs. Another option is to use a thin, hollow needle to remove (aspirate) fluid from the area. If a mass is not a simple cyst (i.e., if it is at least partly solid or it has other concerning features), more imaging tests might be needed to decide if it could be cancer. Some masses can be watched over time with regular mammograms or ultrasound to see if they change, but others may need to be checked with a biopsy. The size, shape, and margins (edges) of the mass can help the radiologist decide how likely it is to be cancer.

- *Breast Density:* Your mammogram report will also contain an assessment of your breast density. Breast density is based on how fibrous and glandular tissues are distributed in your breast, compared to how much of your breast is made up of fatty tissue. Dense breasts are not abnormal, but they are linked to a higher risk of breast cancer. Dense breast tissue can also make it harder to find cancers on a mammogram. Still, experts do not agree with what other tests, if any, should be done along with mammograms in women with dense breasts who are not otherwise at higher risk for breast cancer (based on gene mutations, breast cancer in the family, or other factors).
- Mammograms are the best breast cancer screening tests medical science have in the recent time. But, mammograms have their limits. For example, they are not 100% accurate in showing if a woman has breast cancer. Mammograms have below various limitations [1–8]:
- *False-Negative Mammogram Looks [4]:* A false-negative mammogram looks normal even though breast cancer is present. A false-positive mammogram looks abnormal even though there is no cancer in the breast. A false-negative mammogram looks normal even though breast cancer is present. Overall, screening mammograms do not find about one in five breast cancers. Women with dense breasts are more likely to get false-negative results. False-negative mammograms can give women a false sense of security, thinking that they do not have breast cancer when in fact they do.
- *False-Positive Mammogram Looks [4]:* A false-positive mammogram looks abnormal even though no cancer is present. Abnormal mammograms often require extra testing (diagnostic mammograms, ultrasound, and sometimes MRI or even a breast biopsy) to find out if the change is cancer. False-positive results are more common in younger women and patients who have dense breasts, have had breast biopsies, have breast cancer in the family, or are taking estrogen. About half of the women getting annual mammograms over 10 years will have a false-positive finding at some point. The odds of a false-positive finding are highest for the first mammogram. Women who have past mammograms available for comparison reduce their odds of a false-positive finding by about 50%. False-positive mammograms can cause anxiety. They can also lead to extra tests to be sure cancer is not there, which costs time and money and maybe even physical discomfort.
- *Mammograms Might Not Be Helpful for All Women:* The value of a screening mammogram depends on a woman's overall health. Finding breast cancer early may not help her live longer if she has other serious or life-threatening health problems, such as serious heart disease or severe kidney, liver, or lung disease. The American Cancer Society's [1] breast cancer screening guidelines emphasize that women with serious health problems or short life expectancies should

discuss with their doctors whether they should continue having mammograms. It is important to know that even though mammograms can often find breast cancers that are too small to be felt, treating a small tumor does not always mean it can be cured. A fast-growing or aggressive cancer might have already spread.

- *Overdiagnosis and Overtreatment:* Screening mammograms can often find invasive breast cancer and ductal carcinoma in situ (DCIS, cancer cells in the lining of breast ducts) that need to be treated. However, it is possible that some of the invasive cancers and DCIS found on mammograms would never grow or spread. Finding and treating cancers that would never cause problems is called overdiagnosis. These cancers are not life-threatening and never would have been found or treated if the woman had not gotten a mammogram. The problem is that doctors cannot tell these cancers from those that will grow and spread. Overdiagnosis leads to some women getting treatment that has not been needed (overtreatment) because cancer never would have caused any problems. Doctors can not always tell which cancers will be life-threatening and which will not ever cause problems. Because of this, all cases are treated. This exposes some women to the side effects of cancer treatment, even though it is not needed. Still, overdiagnosis is not thought to happen very often. There is a wide range of estimates of the percentage of breast cancers that might be overdiagnosed by mammography, but the most credible estimates range from 1% to 10%.
- *Radiation Exposure*: Because mammograms are x-ray tests, they expose the breasts to radiation. The amount of radiation from each mammogram is low, but it can still add up over time.

5.1.2 Breast Ultrasound

Breast ultrasound [9, 10] uses sound waves to make a computer picture of the inside of the breast. It can show certain breast changes, like fluid-filled cysts, which are harder to identify on mammograms. Ultrasound is useful for looking at some breast changes, such as lumps (especially those that can be felt but not seen on a mammogram), or changes in women with dense breast tissue. It also can be used to look at a suspicious area that was seen on a mammogram.

Ultrasound is useful because it can often tell the difference between fluid-filled cysts (which are very unlikely to be cancer) and solid masses (which might need further testing to be sure they're not cancer). Ultrasound can also be used to help guide a biopsy needle into an area so that cells can be taken out and tested for cancer. This can also be done in swollen lymph nodes under the arm. Ultrasound is widely available, easy to have, and does not expose a person to radiation. It also costs less than a lot of other options. A gel is put on the skin of the breast, and a wand-like instrument called a transducer is moved over the skin. The transducer sends out sound waves and picks up the echoes as they bounce off body tissues. The echoes are made into a picture on a computer screen. You might feel some pressure

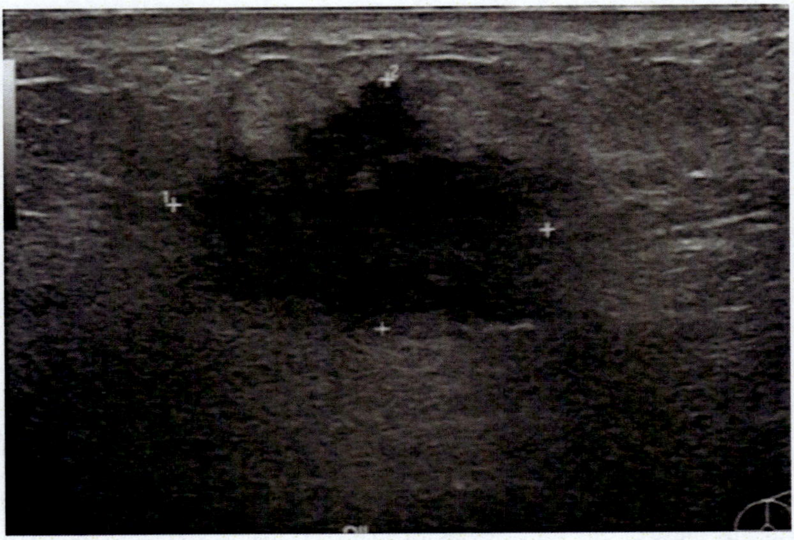

Fig. 5.2 Breast ultrasound image

as the transducer is moved across the breast, but it should not be painful. Automated breast ultrasound (ABUS) is an option that uses a much larger transducer to take hundreds of images that cover nearly the entire breast. When ABUS is done, a second handheld ultrasound is often needed to get more pictures of suspicious areas. A sample ultrasound image of the breast is shown in Fig. 5.2.

5.1.3 *Breast MRI*

Breast MRI (magnetic resonance imaging) [11, 12] uses radio waves and strong magnets to make detailed pictures of the inside of the breast. To help determine the extent of breast cancer, breast MRI is sometimes used in women who already have been diagnosed with breast cancer, to help measure the size of cancer, look for other tumors in the breast, and check for tumors in the opposite breast. But not every woman who has been diagnosed with breast cancer needs a breast MRI. To screen for breast cancer, for certain women at high risk, a screening MRI is recommended along with a yearly mammogram. MRI is not recommended as a screening test by itself because it can miss some cancers that a mammogram would find. Although MRI can find some cancers not seen on a mammogram, it is also more likely to find things that turn out not to be cancer (called a false-positive result). This can result in a woman getting tests and/or biopsies that end up not being needed. This is why MRI is not recommended as a screening test for women at average risk of breast cancer.

- Just as mammograms are done using x-ray machines specially designed for the breasts, breast MRI also requires special equipment. This MRI machine is called an MRI with dedicated breast coils. Not all hospitals and imaging centers have dedicated breast MRI equipment. If you are having a breast MRI, it is important to have it at a facility with dedicated equipment and that can do an MRI-guided breast biopsy (or partners with a facility that can). MRI uses strong magnets instead of radiation to make very detailed, cross-sectional pictures of the body. An MRI scanner takes pictures from many angles as if someone were looking at a slice of your body from the front, from the side, or from above your head. MRI creates pictures of soft tissue parts of the body that would sometimes be hard to see using other imaging tests.
- The most useful MRI exams for breast imaging use a contrast material called gadolinium that is injected into a vein in the arm before or during the exam, which helps to clearly show breast tissue details. (This is not the same as the contrast dye used in CT scans.) It is important to stay very still while the images are being made. Each set of images usually takes a few minutes, and the whole test usually takes between 45 and 60 minutes. After the test, you may be asked to wait while the pictures are checked to see if more is needed.
- A sample breast MR image is shown in Fig. 5.3.

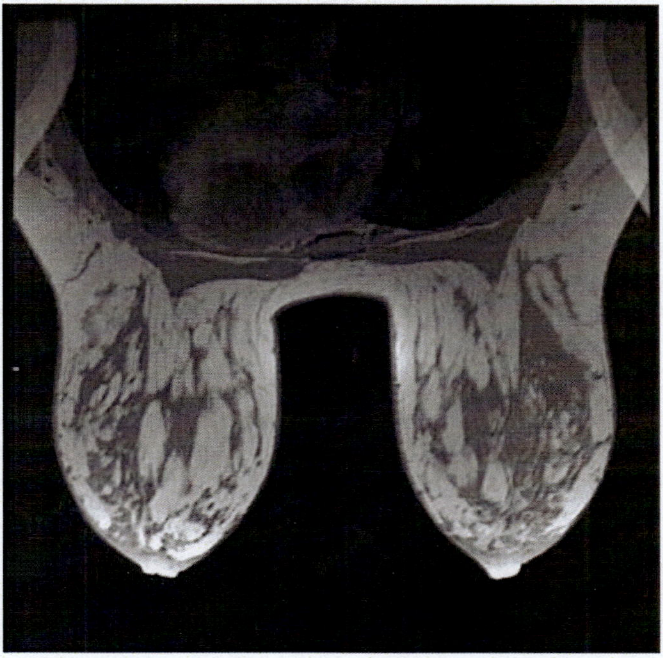

Fig. 5.3 Breast MR image

5.1.4 Newest Imaging Techniques for Detection of Breast Cancer

The most commonly used breast imaging tests at this time are mammograms, ultrasound, and breast MRI. Newer types of tests are now being developed for breast imaging [11–17]. Some of these, such as breast tomosynthesis (3D mammography), are already being used in some centers. Other tests are still being studied, and it will take time to see if they are as good as or better than those used today.

- *Molecular Breast Imaging (MBI)*: Also known as scintimammography or breast specific gamma imaging (BSGI), MBI is a type of nuclear medicine imaging test for the breast. A radioactive chemical is injected into the blood, and a special camera is used to see into the breast. This test is being studied mainly as a way to follow up breast problems (such as a lump or an abnormal mammogram) or to help determine the extent of breast cancer that has already been diagnosed. It can also be used along with mammograms to look for cancer in women with dense breasts. One potential drawback is that it exposes the whole body to radiation, so it is unlikely that this test would be used for screening every year.
- *Positron Emission Mammography (PEM)*: It is a newer imaging test of the breast that is very similar to a PET scan. A form of sugar attached to a radioactive particle is injected into the blood to detect cancer cells. A PEM scan may be better able to detect small clusters of cancer cells within the breast. Right now, it is being studied mainly in women with breast cancer to see if it can help determine the extent of cancer. As with MBI, it exposes the whole body to radiation, so it is unlikely to be a test that could be used every year for breast cancer screening.
- *Contrast-Enhanced Mammography (CEM)*: It is also known as contrast-enhanced spectral mammography (CESM), which is a newer test in which a contrast dye containing iodine is injected into a vein a few minutes before two sets of mammograms (using different energy levels) are taken. The contrast can help the x-rays show any abnormal areas in the breasts. This test can be used to get a better look at areas that appear abnormal on a standard mammogram or to help assess the extent of a tumor in women just diagnosed with breast cancer. Studies are now comparing it to breast MRI in these settings, as well as its possible use in screening women with dense breasts. If it proves to be as good as MRI, CEM could become more widely used because it is quicker to do and is less expensive than MRI.
- *Optical Imaging*: It tests by passing light into the breast and then measures the light that returns or passes through the tissue. The technique does not use radiation and does not require breast compression. Ongoing studies are now looking at combining optical imaging with other tests like MRI, ultrasound, or 3D mammography to help look for breast cancer.
- *Electrical Impedance Tomography (EIT):* It scans the breast for electrical conductivity. It is based on the idea that breast cancer cells conduct electricity differently from normal cells. The test passes a very small electrical current through

the breast and then detects it on the skin of the breast. This is done using small electrodes that are taped to the skin. EIT does not use radiation or compress the breasts. This test can be used to help classify tumors found on mammograms. But at this time, there has not been enough clinical testing to use it for breast cancer screening.

- *Elastography*: A test can be done as part of an ultrasound exam. It is based on the idea that breast cancers tend to be firmer and stiffer than the surrounding breast tissue. For this test, the breast is compressed slightly, and the ultrasound can show how firm a suspicious area is. This test might prove to be useful in telling if the area is more likely to be cancer or a benign (non-cancerous) tumor.

5.2 Various Stages for Detection and Diagnosis of Breast Cancer

In recent times, many problems in healthcare are effectively solved by digital image processing techniques. These techniques improve the quality of images for better understanding and interpretation of humans and improve the quality of images for automatic understanding and interpretation by the machine [18, 19]. In the computer-aided diagnosis system, first medical images are collected, and then preprocessing, segmentation, extraction of features, and, eventually, classifications are performed [20, 21]. Figure 5.4 shows various stages of breast cancer detection and diagnosis system using image processing techniques and artificial intelligence-based classifiers [18].

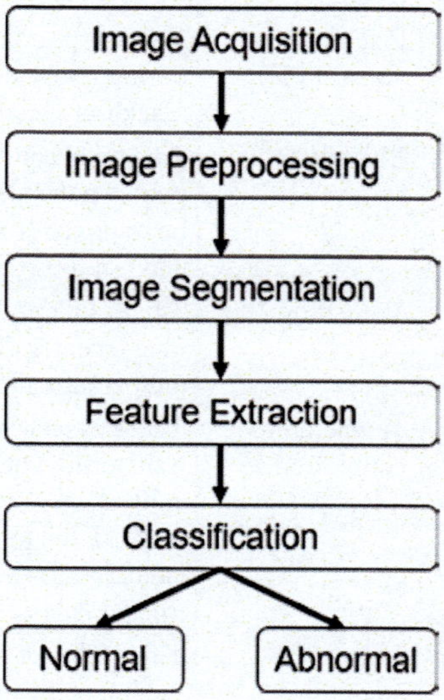

Fig. 5.4 Stages of breast cancer detection and diagnosis system

5.2.1 Breast Image Acquisition

The first step of this system is to acquire a breast image. In this step, various breast data in terms of images are collected from the hospitals. The images are in various formats and probably in a gray map. The DICOM formats of the breast images are used.

5.2.2 Breast Image Preprocessing

The next stage of the system is to preprocess input breast images to improve its quality in terms of removing noise, contrast enhancement, etc. The image preprocessing can be done through various techniques such as filtering, contrast stretching, histogram equalization, etc. Some of the important preprocessing techniques are summarized and discussed in Table 5.1 [18, 22].

This data are collected from the references [18, 22].

5.2.3 Breast Image Preprocessing

The next stage of the system is to preprocess input breast images to improve its quality in terms of removing noise, contrast enhancement, etc. The image preprocessing can be done through various techniques such as filtering, contrast stretch-

Table 5.1 Various image preprocessing techniques

Preprocessing technique	Description
Fixed pattern noise (FPN)	Noise appears in this image due to radiation coming from various detectors during image acquisition. This noise can be eliminated by subtracted blackbody images from the acquired image
Bad pixels	This pixel can be defined as a pixel whose behavior is different from the other pixels in the array. This pixel does not have any useful information and should be removed from the array. The system knows the location of these bad pixels and remove it by the average values of the neighboring pixels
Vignetting	This is one of the noises that cause a darkening of the image corners to the image center due to limited exposure. It depends on both pixel location and temperature difference to the ambient
Temperature calibration	The grayscale values of the image provided by the infrared camera are transformed on a linear scale such as temperature value. The procedure for calibration of temperature was proposed by Ghoncheh et al. [23]. In this method, the put IR camera with reference temperature with various other cameras. As the reference temperature changes, the IR camera captures the image
Noise smoothing	This is one of the famous preprocessing techniques, which eliminates noise in the image by using various types of image processing filters

ing, histogram equalization, etc. Some of the important preprocessing techniques are summarized and discussed in Table 5.2 [18, 24]. These data are collected from references [18, 24].

5.2.4 *Feature Extraction of Breast Tissue*

The transformation of an image into data values is called feature extraction. There are many methodologies to extract or choose features from the image. Some of the most common features are spatial, transform, edges and boundary, color, shape, texture, etc. [21, 25]. These features play a very important role in the diagnosis of breast cancer. Features of the cancer tissue are different from the features of the normal tissue in the breast. These features are capable of dividing normal tissue and abnormal tissue in the breast [21, 25]. Table 5.3 gives some of the most important features that are used for the diagnosis of breast cancer [21, 25].

5.2.5 *Classification of Breast Cancer*

After the extraction of features from the breast tissue, the classification of tissue can be performed with the help of a classifier. The classifier is an artificial intelligence-based algorithm. Various classifiers such as support vector machine (SVM) [26–30], artificial neural network (ANN) [31, 32], k-nearest neighbors (k-NN) [33], and

Table 5.2 Various image segmentation techniques

Segmentation technique	How the technique works	Advantages	Limitations
Edge Detection	Identifies discontinuity in images in terms of edges	Simple and easy to understand	Not good and suitable for images which have undefined edges in it
Thresholding	Used to improve the quality of images in terms of contrast	Easy to apply on any image without prior knowledge of it	Not good and suitable for images that have unclear grayscale values
Region-dependent	Used to identify the area in an image which has similarities in nature	Eliminates noise in the images and improves the quality of images	Complex method and time-consuming; region identification depends on the selection of base pixel information
Fuzzy logic-based method	Used various mathematics properties and rules of fuzzy inference	Used to identify low-level details in the images	Difficult of design, generalized fuzzy function; complex method
Neural network-based method	Used for clustering and classification	Easy to develop	Requires a lot of time for training

Table 5.3 Important features of breast tissues

Mean	Skewness	Entropy (e.g., average entropy, sum entropy)
Standard deviation	Correlation	Variance
Kurtosis	Local binary pattern	Regularity
Contrast	Tissue depth	Difference variance

Table 5.4 Performance of various classifiers for diagnosis of breast cancer

Classifiers	Used breast images	Used features	Range of accuracy (%)	Range of sensitivity (%)	Range of specificity (%)
SVM [26–30]	Mammogram, ultrasound, and thermal	Correlation, entropy, mean, variance, probability, gray level co-occurrence matrix (GLCM) features, LBP features, wavelet features	88.10 to 95.85	81.82 to 97.82	89.09 to 100
Artificial neural network [31, 32]	Mammogram	Age, mean, variance, entropy, contrast, autocorrelation, the maximum probability	67.8 to 92.8	Not reported	Not reported
K-nearest neighbors (k-NN) [29, 33]	Mammogram	Contrast, correlation, entropy, difference variance, maximum probability, GLCM features, gray-level run length matrix (GLRLM) features, Laws texture energy measures (LTEM) features	64 to 92.5	72.2 to 100	54.4 to 87.0
Naïve Bayes [34]	Thermal image	Contrast, correlation, entropy, difference variance, the maximum probability	80.0	76.9	85.7

naïve Bayes [34] are available in the literature and are used for classification of the breast tissue in terms of normal tissue or abnormal tissue. Out of most classifiers the support vector machine is widely used for this purpose [21]. The performance of various classifiers and their advantages and accuracy for the diagnosis of breast cancer are summarized in Table 5.4 [21].

References

1. Breast Cancer Early Detection and Diagnosis. (2016). Weblink: https://www.cancer.org/cancer/breast-cancer/screening-tests-and-early-detection.html. Last Access: May 2020.
2. Radiological Society of North America (RSNA), Mammography (2019). Weblink: https://www.radiologyinfo.org/en/info.cfm?pg=mammo. Last Access: May 2020.

3. Helvie, M. A., & Patterson, S. K. (2014). Chapter 11: Imaging analysis: Mammography. In J. R. Harris, M. E. Lippman, M. Morrow, & C. K. Osborne (Eds.), *Diseases of the breast* (5th ed.). Philadelphia, PA: Lippincott Williams & Wilkins.
4. Hubbard, R. A., Kerlikowske, K., Flowers, C. I., Yankaskas, B. C., Zhu, W., & Miglioretti, D. L. (2011). Cumulative probability of false-positive recall or biopsy recommendation after 10 years of screening mammography: A cohort study. *Annals of Internal Medicine, 155*(8), 481–492.
5. Lee, C. I., & Elmore, J. G. (2014). Chapter 10: Breast cancer screening. In J. R. Harris, M. E. Lippman, M. Morrow, & C. K. Osborne (Eds.), *Diseases of the breast* (5th ed.). Philadelphia, PA: Lippincott Williams & Wilkins.
6. Puliti, D., Duffy, S. W., Miccinesi, G., De Koning, H., Lynge, E., Zappa, M., et al. (2012). Overdiagnosis in mammographic screening for breast cancer in Europe: A literature review. *Journal of Medical Screening, 19*(1_suppl), 42–56.
7. Rosenberg, R. D., Hunt, W. C., Williamson, M. R., Gilliland, F. D., Wiest, P. W., Kelsey, C. A., et al. (1998). Effects of age, breast density, ethnicity, and estrogen replacement therapy on screening mammographic sensitivity and cancer stage at diagnosis: A review of 183,134 screening mammograms in Albuquerque, New Mexico. *Radiology, 209*(2), 511–518.
8. Lauby-Secretan, B., Scoccianti, C., Loomis, D., Benbrahim-Tallaa, L., Bouvard, V., Bianchini, F., et al. (2015). Breast-cancer screening—Viewpoint of the IARC working group. *New England Journal of Medicine, 372*(24), 2353–2358.
9. Esserman, L. J., & Joe, B. N. (2012). *Diagnostic evaluation of women with suspected breast cancer*. Weblink: www.uptodate.com/contents/diagnostic-evaluation-ofwomen-with-suspected-breast-cancer. Last Access: May 2020.
10. Sedgwick, E. (2014). L., chapter 11: Imaging analysis: Ultrasonography. In J. R. Harris, M. E. Lippman, M. Morrow, & C. K. Osborne (Eds.), *Diseases of the breast* (5th ed.). Philadelphia, PA: Lippincott Williams & Wilkins.
11. Slanetz, P. J. (2019). *MRI of the breast and emerging technologies*. Weblink: https://www.uptodate.com/contents/mri-of-the-breast-and-emerging-technologies. Last Access: May 2020.
12. Weinstein, S. P., & Roth, S. O. (2014). Chapter 12: Imaging analysis: Magnetic resonance imaging. In J. R. Harris, M. E. Lippman, M. Morrow, & C. K. Osborne (Eds.), *Diseases of the breast* (5th ed.). Philadelphia, PA: Lippincott Williams & Wilkins.
13. Caldarella, C., Treglia, G., & Giordano, A. (2014). Diagnostic performance of dedicated positron emission mammography using fluorine-18-fluorodeoxyglucose in women with suspicious breast lesions: A meta-analysis. *Clinical Breast Cancer, 14*(4), 241–248.
14. Jochelson, M. (2014). S., chapter 13: Imaging analysis: New breast imaging techniques. In J. R. Harris, M. E. Lippman, M. Morrow, & C. K. Osborne (Eds.), *Diseases of the Breast. 5th ed.* Philadelphia, PA: Lippincott Williams & Wilkins.
15. Perry, H., Phillips, J., Dialani, V., Slanetz, P. J., Fein-Zachary, V. J., Karimova, E. J., et al. (2019). Contrast-enhanced mammography: A systematic guide to interpretation and reporting. *American Journal of Roentgenology, 212*(1), 222–231.
16. Rhodes, D. J., Hruska, C. B., Phillips, S. W., Whaley, D. H., & O'Connor, M. K. (2011). Dedicated dual-head gamma imaging for breast cancer screening in women with mammographically dense breasts. *Radiology, 258*(1), 106–118.
17. Weigert, J. M., Bertrand, M. L., Lanzkowsky, L., Stern, L. H., & Kieper, D. A. (2012). Results of a multicenter patient registry to determine the clinical impact of breast-specific gamma imaging, a molecular breast imaging technique. *American Journal of Roentgenology, 198*(1), W69–W75.
18. Sadoughi, F., Kazemy, Z., Hamedan, F., Owji, L., Rahmanikatigari, M., & Azadboni, T. (2018). Artificial intelligence methods for the diagnosis of breast cancer by image processing: A review. *Breast Cancer: Targets and Therapy, 10*, 219.
19. Kumar, A., & Shaik, F. (2015). *Image processing in diabetic-related causes*. Springer.

20. Haddadnia, J., Hashemian, M., & Hassanpour, K. (2012). Diagnosis of breast cancer using a combination of genetic algorithm and artificial neural network in medical infrared thermal imaging. *Iranian Journal of Medical Physics, 9*(4), 265–274.
21. Pradeep, N., Girisha, H., Sreepathi, B., & Karibasappa, K. (2012). Feature extraction of mammograms. *International Journal of Bioinformatics Research, 4*(1), 241–244.
22. Ibarra-Castanedo, C., Bendada, A., & Maldague, X. (2007, October). Thermographic image processing for NDT. In *IV Conferencia Panamericana de END* (Vol. 79, pp. 1–12).
23. Ghoncheh, M., Pournamdar, Z., & Salehiniya, H. (2016). Incidence and mortality and epidemiology of breast cancer in the world. *Asian Pacific Journal of Cancer Prevention, 17*(S3), 43–46.
24. Sonawane, M. S., & Dhawale, C. A. (2015). A brief survey of image segmentation methods. *International Journal of Computer Applications, 975*, 8887.
25. Lin, H. C., Chiu, C. Y., & Yang, S. N. (2003). Finding textures by textual descriptions, visual examples, and relevance feedback. *Pattern Recognition Letters, 24*(14), 2255–2267.
26. Francis, S. V., Sasikala, M., & Saranya, S. (2014). Detection of breast abnormality from thermograms using curvelet transform based feature extraction. *Journal of Medical Systems, 38*(4), 23.
27. Prabusankarlal, K. M., Thirumoorthy, P., & Manavalan, R. (2015). Assessment of combined textural and morphological features for diagnosis of breast masses in ultrasound. *Human-centric Computing and Information Sciences, 5*(1), 12.
28. Shi, X., Cheng, H., & Hu, L. (2006, October). Mass detection and classification in breast ultrasound images using fuzzy SVM. In *The 9th Joint International Conference on Information Sciences (JCIS-06)*. Atlantis: Press.
29. Basheer, N. M., & Mohammed, M. H. (2013). Classification of breast masses in digital mammograms using support vector machines. *International Journal of Advanced Research in Computer Science and Software Engineering, 3*(10).
30. Acharya, U. R., Ng, E. Y. K., Tan, J. H., & Sree, S. V. (2012). Thermography based breast cancer detection using texture features and support vector machine. *Journal of Medical Systems, 36*(3), 1503–1510.
31. Saini, S., & Vijay, R. (2015, April). Mammogram analysis using feed-forward backpropagation and cascade-forward back propagation artificial neural network. In *2015 fifth international conference on communication systems and network technologies* (pp. 1177–1180). IEEE.
32. Saini, S., & Vijay, R. (2014). Optimization of artificial neural network breast Cancer detection system based on image registration techniques. *International Journal of Computer Applications, 105*(14), 26–29.
33. Ali, M. A., Sayed, G. I., Gaber, T., Hassanien, A. E., Snasel, V., & Silva, L. F. (2015, September). Detection of breast abnormalities of thermograms based on a new segmentation method. In *2015 Federated conference on computer science and information systems (FedCSIS)* (pp. 255–261). IEEE.
34. Milosevic, M., Jankovic, D., & Peulic, A. (2014). Thermography based breast cancer detection using texture features and minimum variance quantization. *EXCLI Journal, 13*, 1204.

Chapter 6
Deep Learning Model for Classification of Breast Cancer

In previous chapters, we discussed the usage of AI in healthcare, medical imaging, and detection of breast cancer with various points. In this chapter, various image datasets for the detection of breast cancer are discussed. Also, the deep learning model for the classification of breast cancer and its performance are presented in this chapter.

6.1 Various Breast Cancer Imaging Datasets

In recent times, computer-aided detection and diagnosis (CAD) systems have been used for the detection and diagnosis of breast cancer. The dataset of various breast mammographic images plays an important role in the development of improving versions of CAD systems. There are many mammographic datasets available in the literature [1] which are presented in this section. Several popular breast cancer datasets such as MIAS, DDSM, and BancoWeb LAPIMO along with other breast cancer datasets are presented and discussed in this section. These datasets are used in many research projects and studied in most of the literature [1]. The details of these datasets are summarized in Tables 6.1 and 6.2 [1–10].

6.1.1 Mammographic Image Analysis Society (MIAS) Digital Mammogram Dataset

This mammogram dataset is the oldest breast cancer image dataset widely used for research and study [2]. This dataset is available at http://peipa.essex.ac.uk/info/mias.html and consists of 320 digital mediolateral-oblique (MLO) images of 161 cases with all types of findings, including abnormal breast images with benign and

K. Shaikh et al., *Artificial Intelligence in Breast Cancer Early Detection and Diagnosis*, https://doi.org/10.1007/978-3-030-59208-0_6

Table 6.1 Popular breast cancer datasets

Parameters	Inbreast [1]	BancoWeb LAPIMO Dataset [4]	DDSM Dataset [3]	MIAS Dataset [2]
Country	Portugal	Brazil	USA	UK
Development year	2008 to 2010	2010	1999	1994
Number of cases	115	320	2620	161
Number of images	410	1400	10,480	322
Views of image	MLO and CC	MLO, CC, and others	MLO and CC	MLO
Type of image	DICOM	TIFF	LJPEG	PGM
Acquisition technique	Screen film	Screen film	Screen film	Screen film
Resolution	14 bits/pixel	12 bits/pixel	8 or 16 bits/pixel	8 bits/pixel
Lesion-type	All kinds	All kinds	All kinds	All kinds
Availability of ground truth	Yes	Yes	Yes	Yes
Availability of BI-RADS annotations	Yes	Yes	Yes	No
Availability of information on breast density	Yes (as per ACR annotations)	Yes (as per ACR annotations)	Yes (as per ACR annotations)	Yes (but not as per ACR annotations)
Easy access	Yes	Yes	Yes	Yes

malign lesions and also normal images. Images in this dataset contain informatio on breast density but not classified as per standards of the American College o Radiology (ACR) [1].

6.1.2 Digital Dataset for Screening Mammography (DDSM)

Digital Dataset is the most usable dataset. Information for this dataset is available a http://www.eng.usf.edu/cvprg/Mammography/Database.html [3]. It is the larges public breast dataset with 10,480 images of 2620 cases, including two images suc as mediolateral-oblique (MLO) and craniocaudal (CC) views from each breast wit all types of findings, including abnormal breast images with benign and malig lesions and also normal images. This dataset has breast density, ACR annotations and Breast Imaging Reporting and Data System (BI-RADS) annotations. Thes annotations give a pixel-level boundary of the image findings [1].

Table 6.2 Other breast cancer datasets

Parameters	Nijmegen [5]	Trueta [6]	IRMA [7]
Country	Netherlands	Spain	Germany
Development year	1998	2008	2008
Number of cases	21	89	Not reported
Number of images	40	320	10,509
Views of image	MLO and CC	MLO and CC	MLO and CC
Type of image	Not reported	DICOM	Various formats
Acquisition technique	Screen film	Full-field digital mammography (FFDM)	Screen film
Resolution	12 bits/pixel	12 bits/pixel	Various bits/pixel
Lesion type	MCCs	All kinds	All kinds
Availability of ground truth	Yes	Yes	Yes
Availability of BI-RADS annotations	Not reported	Yes	Yes
Availability of information on breast density	Not reported	Yes (as per ACR annotations)	Yes (as per ACR annotations)
Easy access	No	No	No
Parameters	**MIRAcle** [8]	**LLNL** [7]	**Malaga** [6]
Country	Greece	USA	Spain
Development year	2009	Unspecified	Unspecified
Number of cases	196	50	35
Number of images	204	198	Unspecified
Views of image	Unspecified	MLO and CC	MLO and CC
Type of image	Unspecified	Image cytometry standard (ICS)	Raw
Acquisition technique	Unspecified	Unspecified	Unspecified
Resolution	Unspecified	12 bits/pixel	12 bits/pixel
Lesion type	Unspecified	Calcifications	Masses
Availability of ground truth	Yes	Yes	Yes
Availability of BI-RADS annotations	Yes	Unspecified	Unspecified
Availability of information on breast density	No	Unspecified	Unspecified
Easy access	Limited (2011)	Paid	Unspecified

6.1.3 BancoWeb LAPIMO Dataset

BancoWeb LAPIMO Dataset is a new and recently developed dataset. Information is available after registration on this Weblink: http://lapimo.sel.eesc.usp.br/bancoweb/ [4]. This dataset contains 1473 breast images of 320 cases with MLO, CC, and magnification views of normal breast images and abnormal images with benign and malign findings. Patient information with BI-RADS annotations is available in this dataset.

6.1.4 *Other Breast Cancer Datasets*

Other breast cancer datasets such as Nijmegen [5], Trueta [6], Image Retrieval in Medical Applications (IRMA) [7], MIRAcle [8], Lawrence Livermore National Laboratory (LLNL) [7], and Malaga [6] are available in the literature. These datasets are not famous and not used worldwide. These datasets are used for other types of studies at the country level. The details of these datasets are summarized in Table 6.2. Also, Magic-5 [9], which was previously known as GPCALMA, is an Italian database built in 2002. This contains 967 cases with 3369 images in different views such as MLO, CC, and lateral. The resolution of these images is 12 bits/pixels, saved in the Digital Imaging and Communication in Medicine (DICOM) format. The limitation of this dataset is related to the different acquisition environments which makes it very heterogeneous [1]. MammoGrid [10] was developed by a collaboration between the United Kingdom, Italy, and Switzerland. The images of the dataset are saved in the DICOM format. The main limitation of this dataset is that it has limited access to specific institutions in Europe.

6.2 Evaluation Parameters for Performance of Classification Model

Diagnostic breast images are classified using various types of machine learning (ML) and deep learning (DL) algorithms in several ways depending on the types of images, patients, diseases, and the types of hospitals. The performance of classifiers is measured by quality parameters such as sensitivity, specificity, and accuracy of classifiers [11]. Sensitivity gives the probability that the classification test has a positive value (i.e., the patient has breast cancer). Specificity gives the probability that the classification test has a negative value (i.e., the patient has no breast cancer). Accuracy gives the probability that the classification of breast cancer test is correctly performed. The equations for these three parameters are given as [11]

$$\text{Sensitivity} = \frac{\text{TP}}{\text{TP} + \text{FN}} \tag{6.1}$$

$$\text{Specificity} = \frac{\text{TN}}{\text{TN} + \text{FP}} \tag{6.2}$$

$$\text{Accuracy} = \frac{\text{TP} + \text{TN}}{\text{TP} + \text{TN} + \text{FP} + \text{FN}} \tag{6.3}$$

where *TP* gives correctly classified positive values, *TN* gives correctly classified negative values, *FP* gives incorrectly classified positive values, and *FN* gives incorrectly classified negative values.

6.3 Deep Learning Model for Classification of Breast Cancer

In this section, the performance of the convolutional neural network (CNN)-based deep learning model is presented and discussed for the classification of breast cancer. The performance of the model is measured with the help of the mini-MIAS mammogram dataset [12]. This dataset contains 321 breast images where 211 images are normal and 110 images have some cancer tissue in it. For the evaluation of classifier algorithms, this dataset divides into three different datasets such as training, validation, and test. The training dataset contains 225 images, the validation dataset contains 48 images, and the test dataset contains 48 images. The sample images of this dataset are shown in Fig. 6.1. The selection of these datasets is done by a random manner, and cross-fold validation is used for validation of the model.

The CNN model for the classification of breast cancer images is shown in Fig. 6.2. This model contains seven convolutional layers along with max-pooling for the extraction of features from the input images. After extraction of features,

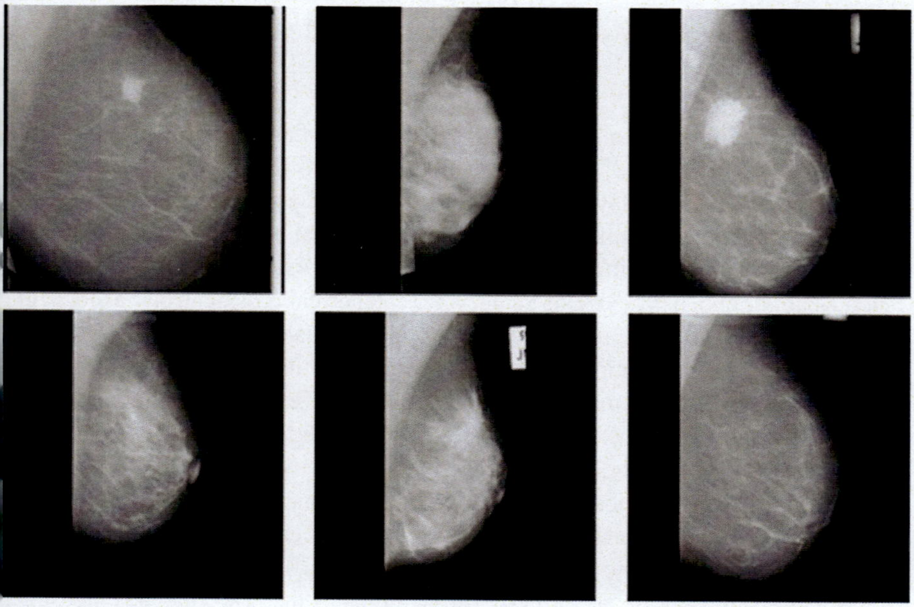

Fig. 6.1 Sample breast images of mini-MIAS dataset

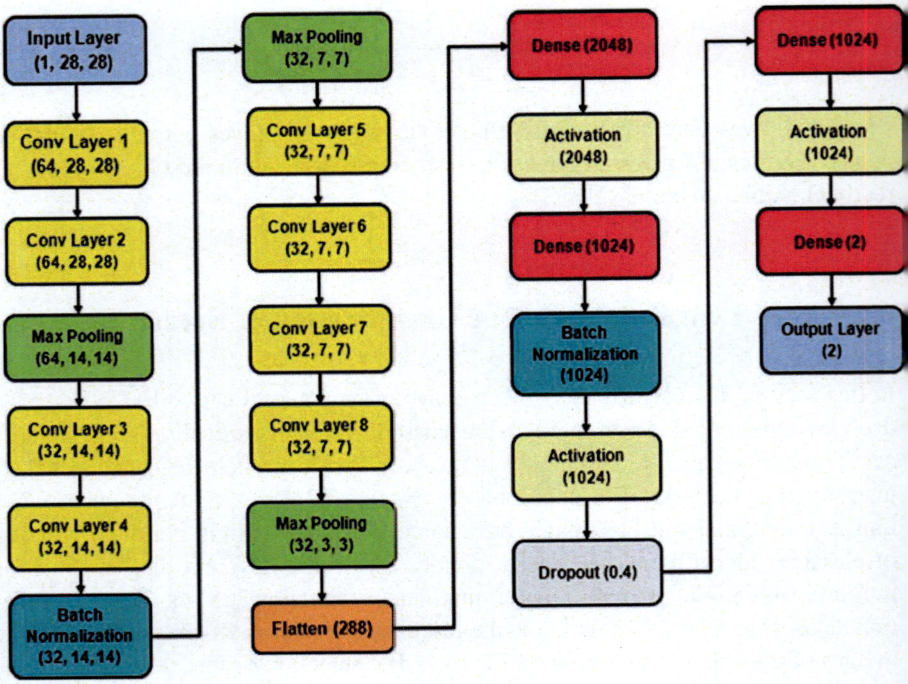

Fig. 6.2 CNN model for classification of breast cancer

Fig. 6.3 Confusion matrix for performance evaluation of CNN model

		Predicated Values	
		Normal	Abnormal
Actual Values	Normal	TP	FP
	Abnormal	FN	TN

these features convert into a vector with the help of a flattened layer and give as a input of a neural network. This neural network contains three hidden layers and on output layer. The output layer of this network contains a softmax function that clas sifies input images as normal breast image or abnormal breast image.

The training and testing of the CNN model can use various hyperparameter such as no. of epoch = 5, size of batch = 32, categorical cross-entropy as loss func tion, stochastic gradient descent (SGD) optimizer, and tenfold cross-validatio along with different learning rates. After training and testing of models, the belo confusion matrix is summarized, which gives many evaluation parameter value such as true-positive, true-negative, false-positive, and false-negative. The confu sion matrix is given in Fig. 6.3.

In Fig. 6.3, the true-positive indicates that a woman has no breast cancer, bu models predict the woman has no breast cancer in this case. The false-positive ind cates that a woman has no breast cancer, but the model predicts that a woman ha breast cancer in this case. The true-negative indicates that a woman has breast car cer, but the model predicts that a woman has cancer in this case. The false-negativ

Table 6.3 Confusion matrix and performance of CNN model for various learning rates

Learning rate	Confusion matrix	Accuracy (%)	Sensitivity (%)	Specificity (%)
0.001	$\begin{bmatrix} & N & ABN & Total \\ N & 32 & 10 & 42 \\ ABN & 5 & 1 & 6 \\ Total & 37 & 11 & 48 \end{bmatrix}$	68.75	76.19	86.48
0.01	$\begin{bmatrix} & N & ABN & Total \\ N & 41 & 1 & 42 \\ ABN & 6 & 0 & 6 \\ Total & 47 & 1 & 48 \end{bmatrix}$	85.41	97.61	87.23
0.1	$\begin{bmatrix} & N & ABN & Total \\ N & 42 & 0 & 42 \\ ABN & 6 & 0 & 6 \\ Total & 48 & 0 & 48 \end{bmatrix}$	87.50	100	87.50

where N = normal and ABN = abnormal.

Table 6.4 Comparative comparison of presented CNN model with existing models

Researcher	No. of breast cancer images	Used algorithms	Accuracy (%)
Listgarten et al. (2004) [13]	174	SVM, NB, and decision tree	69, 67, and 68
Park et al. (2014) [14]	189	Graph-based semi-supervised learning (GSSL), TSVM, SVM, NB, and RF	72.5, 54.3, 52.8, 59.2, and 66.4
Sountharrajan et al. (2017) [15]	198	SVM, NB, and C4.5 decision tree	79.25, 77.25, and 77.25
Presented deep learning model	321	CNN	87.50

indicates that a woman has breast cancer, but the model predicts the woman has no breast cancer in this case. The confusion matrix for various learning rates along with other evaluation parameters is summarized in Table 6.3. Referring to Table 6.3, the maximum accuracy of the classification of breast cancer images can achieve up to 87.5%, while maximum sensitivity is 100% along with maximum specificity which is 87.5%.

Table 6.4 shows a comparative analysis of the presented CNN model along with other existing models available in the literature. The existing models are developed with the help of conventional machine learning algorithms such as support vector machine (SVM), decision tree (DT), naïve Bayes, and random forest. The maximum accuracy of existing models can be achieved by up to 79.25 % for the classification of breast cancer images, while the presented CNN model gives the accuracy of up to 87.5 % for this purpose.

References

1. Moreira, I. C., Amaral, I., Domingues, I., Cardoso, A., Cardoso, M. J., & Cardoso, J. S. (2012) In breast: Toward a full-field digital mammographic database. *Academic Radiology, 19*(2) 236–248.
2. Suckling, J. P. (1994). *The mammographic image analysis society digital mammogram database*. Digital Mammo, 375–386.
3. Netsch, T., & Peitgen, H. O. (1999). Scale-space signatures for the detection of clusterec microcalcifications in digital mammograms. *IEEE Transactions on Medical Imaging, 18*(9) 774–786.
4. Matheus, B. R. N., & Schiabel, H. (2011). Online mammographic images database for development and comparison of CAD schemes. *Journal of Digital Imaging, 24*(3), 500–506.
5. Lo, C., S., Chung, P., C., Chang, C., I. (1996). A computerized system for detection an segmentation of clustered microcalcifications. Joint Conference of International Compute Symposium 1996; 247–253.
6. Oliver, I., & Malagelada, A. (2007). *Automatic mass segmentation in mammographic images* Universitat de Girona.
7. Oliveira, J. E., Gueld, M. O., Araújo, A. D. A., Ott, B., & Deserno, T. M. (2008, March) Toward a standard reference database for computer-aided mammography. In *Medical imagin 2008: Computer-aided diagnosis* (Vol. 6915, p. 69151Y). International Society for Optics an Photonics.
8. Antoniou, Z. C., Giannakopoulou, G. P., Andreadis, I. I., Nikita, K. S., Ligomenides, P. A., & Spyrou, G. M. (2009, November). A web-accessible mammographic image database dedicate to combined training and evaluation of radiologists and machines. In *2009 9th Internationa conference on information technology and applications in biomedicine* (pp. 1–4). IEEE.
9. Tangaro, S., Bellotti, R., De Carlo, F., Gargano, G., Lattanzio, E., Monno, P., et al. (2008) MAGIC-5: An Italian mammographic database of digitised images for research. *La radiologiamedica, 113*(4), 477–485.
10. Warren, R., Solomonides, A. E., Del Frate, C., Warsi, I., Ding, J., Odeh, M., et al. (2007) MammoGrid—A prototype distributed mammographic database for Europe. *Clinica Radiology, 62*(11), 1044–1051.
11. El-Dahshan, E. A., Salem, A. B. M., & Younis, T. H. (2009). A hybrid technique for automati MRI brain images classification. Studia Univ. babes-Bolyai. *Informatica, 54*(1), 55–67.
12. MIAS Mini Mammograms Dataset. (2012). Weblink: http://peipa.essex.ac.uk/info/mias.htm Last Access: May 2020.
13. Listgarten, J., Damaraju, S., Poulin, B., Cook, L., Dufour, J., Driga, A., et al. (2004). Predictiv models for breast cancer susceptibility from multiple single nucleotide polymorphism *Clinical Cancer Research, 10*(8), 2725–2737.
14. Park, C., Ahn, J., Kim, H., & Park, S. (2014). Integrative gene network construction to analyz cancer recurrence using semi-supervised learning. *PLoS One, 9*(1), e86309.
15. Sountharrajan, S., Karthiga, M., Suganya, E., & Rajan, C. (2017). Automatic classification biomedical prognosis of invasive breast cancer. *Asian Pacific J Cancer Prevent APJCP, 18*(9 2541.

Index

K. Shaikh et al., *Artificial Intelligence in Breast Cancer Early Detection and Diagnosis*, https://doi.org/10.1007/978-3-030-59208-0

U

V

X

Asbestos Disaster